INTRODUCTION TO
CLINICAL EXAMINATION

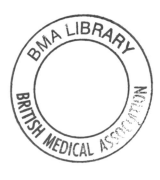

For Elsevier
Commissioning Editor: Laurence Hunter
Project Development Manager: Helen Leng
Project Manager: Nancy Arnott
Designer: Erik Bigland
Illustration Manager: Bruce Hogarth

INTRODUCTION TO

CLINICAL EXAMINATION

Michael J Ford MB ChB(Hons) MD FRCPE
Consultant Physician
Western General Hospital, Edinburgh;
Clinical Sub-Dean and Part-time Senior Lecturer,
Faculty of Medicine, University of Edinburgh

Iain Hennessey MB ChB(Hons) BSc(Hons)
Senior House Officer
A & E Medicine
Royal Infirmary of Edinburgh
Edinburgh

Alan Japp MB ChB(Hons) BSc(Hons)
Senior House Officer
General Medicine
Royal Infirmary of Edinburgh
Edinburgh

Illustrated by **Robert Britton**

EIGHTH EDITION

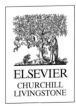

ELSEVIER
CHURCHILL
LIVINGSTONE

EDINBURGH LONDON NEW YORK OXFORD
PHILADELPHIA ST LOUIS SYDNEY TORONTO 2005

ELSEVIER
CHURCHILL LIVINGSTONE

© Harcourt Publishers Limited 2000
© 2005, Elsevier Limited. All rights reserved.

First edition 1974
Second edition 1977
Third edition 1983
Fourth edition 1985
Fifth edition 1989
Sixth edition 1993
Seventh edition 2000

Working together to grow
libraries in developing countries

www.elsevier.com | www.bookaid.org | www.sabre.org

ELSEVIER | BOOK AID International | Sabre Foundation

ISBN 0443074178
International student edition 0443074186

British Library Cataloguing in Publication Data
A catalogue record for this book is available from the British Library

Library of Congress Cataloging in Publication Data
A catalog record for this book is available from the Library of Congress

Note
Medical knowledge is constantly changing. Standard safety precautions must be followed, but as new research and clinical experience broaden our knowledge, changes in treatment and drug therapy may become necessary or appropriate. Readers are advised to check the most current product information provided by the manufacturer of each drug to be administered to verify the recommended dose, the method and duration of administration, and contraindications. It is the responsibility of the practitioner, relying on experience and knowledge of the patient, to determine dosages and the best treatment for each individual patient. Neither the publisher nor the authors assume any liability for any injury and/or damage to persons or property arising from this publication.
The Publisher

ELSEVIER your source for books, journals and multimedia in the health sciences

www.elsevierhealth.com

The publisher's policy is to use **paper manufactured from sustainable forests**

Printed in China

Preface

The most important core skills for medical students to master are history taking and clinical examination. The extensively revised, eighth edition has been written with the philosophy that the acquisition of clinical skills is most effectively undertaken at the bedside. This pocketbook should be used as a companion, to be taken onto the wards and into consulting rooms where the information is most needed.

The book begins with a system of history taking followed by a new chapter on the analysis of key symptoms. The remaining chapters cover the physical examination of each of the major systems, beginning with an overview of the important signs and symptoms. Each stage of the examination starts with a detailed, step-by-step description of the examination method complemented by relevant illustrations, diagrams and tables on the facing page.

This book is intended primarily for use at the outset of clinical training; once students have achieved proficiency in the basic skills of interviewing and examining, the book should also prove useful for revision. More detailed information about clinical method and the related basic clinical sciences can be obtained from textbooks such as 'Macleod's Clinical Examination', Douglas, Nicol, Robertson, 11th edition, 2005, Elsevier Churchill Livingstone or 'Clinical Examination,' Epstein, Perkin, Cookson, de Bono, 3rd edition, 2003, Mosby.

Edinburgh   M.F.
                                                                               I. H.
                                                                               A. J.

Acknowledgements

The authors wish to thank Dr John F Munro, the previous co-author of the book, Dr Graham Douglas, Dr Fiona Nicol and Dr Colin Robertson, co-authors of Macleod's Clinical Examination, 11th edition, and the friends, medical students and colleagues who have given their constructive criticism and advice.

Contents

History taking

Taking a patient's history is the most important skill in medicine; it is the keystone of clinical diagnosis and the foundation for the doctor–patient relationship. The history will help you to formulate a differential diagnosis and focus your physical examination. As important, it will also help you in getting to know patients, winning their confidence and understanding the social context of their illness. The consultation is best viewed as a 'meeting of two experts': the patient, an expert on the experience of illness and the unique context in which it has occurred, and the clinician, an expert on the diagnosis and management of illness.

The aims of history taking are threefold:

- To identify the relevant organ system(s) responsible for symptoms
- To clarify the nature of the pathological processes at play
- To characterize the social context of patients' illness, their concerns, their interpretation of symptoms, beliefs and attributions and any limitations of daily activities consequent upon their illness.

Diagnostic information

The key to reaching an accurate diagnosis is obtaining a detailed description of the patient's symptoms. Every individual symptom suggests a differential diagnosis which may initially be wide ranging but can be brought into sharper focus by obtaining as much detail as possible about the symptomatology. A systematic method of describing symptoms is described in Chapter 2 and can be applied to all symptoms. This information is complemented by assessment of risk factors for the diagnoses under consideration. A risk factor is any piece of information that increases the likelihood of a particular diagnosis, e.g. a past history of recent hip surgery and immobilization greatly increases the diagnostic probability of acute pulmonary embolism in a patient presenting with sudden onset of breathlessness.

Approach to the patient

You will feel intimidated in your first attempts at history taking. Most patients, however, are keen to put the apprehensive student at ease. Aim to develop a professional but friendly manner. View the consultation as a meeting of two experts and you will quickly gain an effective rapport with the patient. Try to be caring and compassionate but remember that you are not directly responsible for your patient's medical care. Show tolerance, particularly with the elderly and the deaf. Seek first to understand and not judge the patient so that you don't react to patients with criticism, anger or dismissal.

Introduce yourself with a friendly greeting, giving your name and status. Explain the purpose of your visit, ask for and remember the patient's name and request permission to interview and examine the patient. Some patients rapidly tire of being questioned or examined, and others may be depressed because they are ill or apprehensive in a strange environment. If there are difficulties in establishing a rapport, try to determine the reason; if in doubt, consult the medical or nursing staff.

Factors in establishing rapport

- Introduce yourself in a warm, friendly manner.
- Maintain good eye contact.
- Listen attentively.
- Facilitate verbally and non-verbally.
- Touch patients appropriately.
- Discuss patients' personal concerns.

Eliciting accurate, detailed and unbiased information from a patient is a skilled task and not simply a matter of recording the patient's responses to a checklist of questions. Adopt a personal, conversational style rather than an interrogative approach and don't confuse patients with medical jargon. Avoid interrupting patients, particularly as they begin to tell you the story of the presenting features of the illness.

Figure 1.1 illustrates a system for gathering information which begins with the patient's own account of events. Given the opportunity, most patients will provide relevant information about their illness and often need to talk about their troubles. Recognizing the patient's need to talk without interruption and being a good listener will greatly help you to establish a good relationship quickly. Try to limit your intervention at this stage to encouraging the flow of information with simple verbal and non-verbal cues but, if necessary, steer the talkative individual from less relevant facts. Clarify any details about which you remain uncertain such as the precise meaning of ambiguous terms, e.g. indigestion. When asking specific questions relating to symptoms, avoid leading questions which might compromise the quality of information obtained. If asking about the aggravating and relieving factors of pain, ask as follows:

- Tell me everything you noticed about the pain.
- Did you notice whether anything made the pain better or worse?
- Did moving around make the pain better, worse or have no effect?

NB: Try to avoid suggesting a particular answer to the patient, such as by asking 'Was the pain worse when you moved?' Once you are satisfied that you have all the necessary information, it is important to summarize the story, as you understand it, so that the patient can check its accuracy and alter or add to it if required.

Some patients may be unable to give a history because they are too ill, confused, demented or unconscious. It is then vital to obtain further information from relatives, friends and the patient's general practitioner.

Listen

Allow patients to tell the story in their own words
Encourage their flow with verbal and non-verbal cues
Try not to interrupt

Clarify

Exact nature of vague terms or lay terms
Timing of events
Apparent inconsistencies or gaps in the story

Question

Specific areas of relevance
Use open questions initially
Avoid leading questions

Summarise

Outline the story as you understand it
Invite patient to correct inaccuracies

Fig. 1.1 System for gathering information.

1.1 Top ten technique tips
1. Give the patient your undivided attention
2. Keep your note-taking to a minimum when the patient is talking
3. Use language which the patient can understand
4. Let patients tell their own story in their own way
5. Steer patients towards the relevant
6. Use open questions initially and specific (closed) questions later
7. Clarify the meaning of any lay terms or diagnoses patients use
8. Remember that the history includes events up to the day of interview
9. Summarize (reflect back) the story for the patient to check
10. Utilize all available sources of information

There is no single, correct way to take a history; with time you will develop your own style; however, one effective and commonly used sequence comprises:

- Introduction
- Presenting complaint
- History of current illness
- Systemic enquiry
- Past medical history
- Drugs and allergies
- Family history
- Social and personal history
- Patient's ideas, concerns and expectations.

Introduction

Introduce yourself to the patient giving your name and status as a student. Ask the patient's name, how he/she prefers to be addressed and ask for permission to take a history and perform a physical examination.

Presenting complaint

Establish the principal symptom or symptoms that caused the patient to seek medical attention, when it first appeared and how it has changed over time.

- What was the main problem that made you want to see the doctor?
- When did you first notice the problem?
- Has the problem changed since it first came on?

Record the presenting complaint in the patient's own words, for example 'a terrible pain in my chest', the date and time of its first occurrence and if the problem has changed in any way since its onset.

The aim is to obtain a chronological account of the relevant events, including interventions and their outcomes and a detailed description of the patient's main symptoms.

Patient's account

As described earlier, you should begin by inviting patients to provide an account of recent events in their own words. Learn to listen without interruption and encourage the patient to continue the story right up to the time of interview.

- When did you last feel fit and well?
- When did you first notice a change in your usual state of health?
- What was the first symptom you noticed?
- When was that and what has happened since?
- What else have you noticed about your health?
- What has happened to you since you came into hospital?
- How do you feel at the moment?

Interrogation

When the patient has completed the story, clarify the description by specific questioning to obtain a detailed chronological account of the development of the illness from the first symptom to the time of the interview. Do not be misled by accepting the patient's interpretations uncritically; for example 'flu' may really be a trivial 'cold' or a serious systemic illness. Identify what investigations and treatment have been undertaken so far and what the patient has been told about the illness. Obtain a detailed description of every symptom reported by the patient using the system outlined in Chapter 2.

Ask about all the cardinal symptoms in each of the major systems (see checklist in Table 1.2 below), using lay terms to broaden the scope, e.g. indigestion. See Chapter 2 for symptom definitions and for further information.

1.2 Checklist of symptoms	
General	**Genitourinary**
Fatigue	Dysuria
Anorexia	Frequency/nocturia
Weight change	Change in colour/smell of urine
Itch	Prostatic symptoms
Rashes	Urethral/vaginal discharge
Low mood	Incontinence
Fevers/night sweats	Menstrual difficulties
Heat/cold intolerance	Postmenstrual bleeding
Change in appearance	Sexual difficulties
Cardiorespiratory	**Central nervous system**
Chest pain	Headaches
Breathlessness	Fits/faints/funny turns
Orthopnoea	Weakness
Paroxysmal nocturnal dyspnoea	Sensory symptoms
Palpitation	Changes in taste/smell
Cough	Hearing disturbance
Sputum	Visual disturbance
Wheeze	Speech disturbance
Haemoptysis	Dizziness
Gastrointestinal	**Locomotor**
Swallowing difficulty	Pain
Nausea and vomiting	Stiffness
Haematemesis	Immobility
Heartburn	Swelling
Indigestion	Loss of joint function
Abdominal pain	
Change in bowel habit	
Change in colour/consistency of motions	

Use a variety of questions to jog the patient's memory. Patients may have forgotten about previous health problems or believe them to be irrelevant or too embarrassing. Ask about the outcome of any previous medical or radiological examinations including those tests performed for employment or insurance purposes. Check the patient's immunization status, e.g. tetanus, rubella and tuberculosis. Ask about any travel or residence abroad, especially if infection is suspected and the cause is not immediately obvious, e.g. falciparum malaria.

Checklist

- Have you had any similar episodes in the past?
- What investigations have you had in the past? X-rays? Scans?
- What were the results of your previous tests?
- Have you had any other medical problems or conditions?
- Have you had any serious illness in the past?
- Have you been in hospital before?
- Have you had any operations?
- Have you ever had a blood transfusion?
- What problems have you seen your GP about in the past?
- What injuries or accidents have you had in the past?
- When and where have you travelled abroad?
- Have you ever had any of the following conditions: asthma/chronic obstructive pulmonary disease (COPD)/angina/heart attack/stroke/diabetes/epilepsy/rheumatic fever/blood clot in the leg or lung/tuberculosis (TB)/jaundice/high blood pressure/high blood cholesterol?

Accurately record the patient's drug therapy including 'over-the-counter' remedies. Adverse drug effects are a common cause of ill health and may explain any worsening of existing symptoms, particularly if drug therapy has changed recently. Always ask patients if they have brought their medications with them and if they carry a list (repeat prescription). If in doubt, check with their GP surgery. Check if the drug therapy has changed recently, if the drugs on the referral letter/repeat prescription match the list of drugs patients actually take and how often they forget to take their tablets. Ask about previous allergies, drug reactions and their nature.

Checklist

- What medications do you actually take?
- What 'over-the-counter' drugs or herbal remedies do you use?
- Do you take low-dose aspirin? Vitamin pills?
- Do you take the oral contraceptive pill? HRT (hormone replacement therapy)?
- Have your medications changed at all recently?
- How often do you forget to take your tablets?
- Have any medicines ever upset you? If so, how?
- What exactly happens when you take that medication?
- Are you allergic to anything? – Hay fever? Asthma? Eczema?

In addition to providing information on any predisposition to disease, the family history may help uncover the patient's underlying and, often unspoken, anxieties. When relevant, draw a family tree to map the inheritance pattern of particular diseases (Fig. 1.2 illustrates an inherited disorder). Use symbols in a pedigree chart beginning with the affected person first found to have the trait (propositus if male, proposita if female); include all the relevant information regarding siblings and all maternal and paternal relatives.

Checklist

- Has any family member suffered from a similar problem?
- Do you know of any illnesses that run in your family?
- Has any member of your family died before the age of 60?

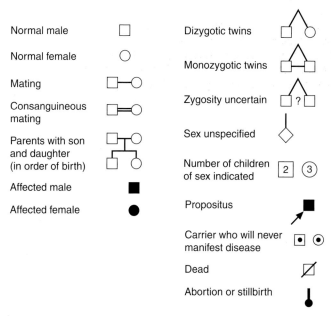

Normal male		Dizygotic twins
Normal female		Monozygotic twins
Mating		Zygosity uncertain
Consanguineous mating		
Parents with son and daughter (in order of birth)		Sex unspecified
		Number of children of sex indicated
Affected male		Propositus
Affected female		Carrier who will never manifest disease
		Dead
		Abortion or stillbirth

Fig. 1.2 Common symbols used in constructing a family tree.

An individual's health and well-being are affected by occupational, social and personal factors. Knowledge of the patient's background is useful, not only for diagnosis but also for management. How patients think, live and behave influence how they cope with illness. The details of patients' personal lives, events and difficulties serve both to inform you and reaffirm your interest in the patient as an individual. Get to know your patients and their concerns; seek to understand the impact of illness on their personal, working and family lives. Ask about their employment, housing, personal and sexual relationships (or lack of them), leisure interests, physical exercise and the use of drugs including tobacco, alcohol and other recreational drugs, e.g. cannabis. Quantify cigarette consumption in pack years (20/day/year), and alcohol consumption as average number of units per week.

Checklist

- What jobs have you done since starting work?
- What did these jobs involve?
- How do you spend your time when you are not at work?
- Where do you live? What is your house like?
- Are you able to do all the activities that you need to be able to do?
- Who lives with you at home? Partner? Single?
- Have you had children? Any worries or illness with them?
- How many sexual partners have you had? Male? Female?
- Have you ever smoked? Ever been a heavy drinker?

1 alcohol unit (8 g) $\equiv$ $\frac{1}{2}$ pint beer $\equiv$ 1 small glass wine $\equiv$ 1 single spirit.

CAGE Questionnaire

C 'Have you felt the need to **c**ut down your alcohol intake?'
A 'Have you felt **a**nnoyed that folk think you drink too much?'
G 'Have you felt **g**uilty about your use of alcohol?'
E 'Have you needed an **e**ye-opener in the morning to feel better?'
(Scores of two or more positive answers indicate a significant alcohol problem.)

The commonest cause of patient dissatisfaction from consultations is a failure of communication. Consultations are significantly more likely to be ranked by patients as 'good consultations' when a doctor asks about the personal aspects of a patient's life, compared with consultations in which this does not occur. If the personal and social history is overlooked, unfounded assumptions may be made regarding patients' understanding of their illnesses, leading to either unnecessary anxiety or unrealistic optimism. Patients cannot be appropriately reassured if their ideas, concerns and expectations are not fully explored. Similarly, patients cannot actively participate in and comply with their treatment if their views have not been heard.

Students can play a useful role in this regard, as patients may confide in them anxieties about their illnesses which they have felt unable to discuss with members of the nursing or medical staff. In such situations, the student should seek the patient's permission to pass on this information to a member of the medical team.

Checklist

- What have you thought might be causing your symptoms?
- Is there anything in particular that concerns you?
- What have you been told about your illness?
- What do you expect to happen while you are in hospital?
- Do you expect any difficulties in coping when you go home?
- Do you have any questions you would like me to pass on to the medical or nursing staff?

Symptoms of disease

'TINA' symptom analysis

The systematic analysis of any symptom is best achieved by a detailed assessment of its **T**iming, **I**nfluences, **N**ature and **A**ssociated features (Tables 2.1 and 2.2).

Timing

The pathological process responsible for a symptom can often be deduced by attention to its timing. As a general principle, vascular processes produce symptoms of sudden onset, inflammatory and infective processes arise over a period of hours, days and weeks, and malignant or degenerative processes arise over months and years. A symptom may either occur as a single episode, multiple episodes or continuously.

Influences

Aggravating and relieving factors affect symptom severity and provide clues to the diagnosis, e.g. the chest pain of angina pectoris is characteristically brought on by exertion and relieved by rest. Potential influences include medical treatment, and you should assess the effect of all therapeutic interventions on symptoms (positive, negative or neutral).

Nature

Ask patients to describe what they are experiencing in as much detail as possible. Find out what patients mean by the terms they use, e.g. 'indigestion', and ask them to describe its features in detail. For any type of pain, identify the main site, radiation, character and severity. Severity may be quantified in many ways, e.g. on a scale of 0–10, comparison with previous illness, impact on activities, walking distance, etc.

Associations

Ask about any other symptoms that may have occurred around the same time. Clarify the timing of symptoms in relation to each other and identify the nature and characteristics of features that consistently preceded or followed the symptom described.

2.1 TINA: elements in assessment

Timing	Onset, duration, pattern, progression
Influences	Precipitating, aggravating and relieving factors
Nature	Character, severity, site, radiation, volume
Associations	Symptoms, relationship

2.2 TINA: assessment questions

Timing
Duration	When was the first time you noticed it?
Onset	What were you doing? How quickly did it appear?
Progression	Has it been the same ever since, getting worse or better?
Pattern	Have you ever had any similar episodes in the past? If so: How many episodes? How often? How long did they last? How long between episodes? Do episodes occur at any particular time of day, week or month? Has the pattern been changing?

Influences
Aggravating	What were you doing when you first noticed it? Have you noticed anything that tends to bring it on? Have you noticed anything that makes it worse?
Relieving	When it is present, is there anything that makes it better? What have you tried to improve it? Did it do any good? Does it help to exercise or take food, drugs or antacids?

Nature
Character	Tell me what it feels like when it comes on? How would you describe it? Does it change in character?
Severity	How much does it affect you? How does it compare with previous episodes? Is it worse than toothache or labour pains? Does it make you sweat, feel squeamish or vomit?

Associations
Symptoms	Is there anything else you notice with these episodes? Have you felt unwell in any other way?
Relationship	Does it occur before, during or after an episode? Is it a constant feature or only on some occasions?

↓	lowered, reduced	ICP	intracranial pressure
↑	raised, increased	IHD	ischaemic heart disease
ΔΔ	differential diagnosis	LMP	last menstrual period
AAA	abdominal aortic aneurysm	LOC	loss of consciousness
		LVF	left ventricular failure
ACE	angiotensin-converting enzyme	MI	myocardial infarction
		MS	multiple sclerosis
Ca	calcium	NSAIDs	non-steroidal anti-inflammatory drugs
CNS	central nervous system		
COPD	chronic obstructive pulmonary disease	OA	osteoarthritis
		OCP	oral contraceptive pill
CSH	carotid sinus hypersensitivity	PE	pulmonary embolism
		PID	pelvic inflammatory disease
CVA	cerebrovascular accident		
DHx	drug history	PMHx	past medical history
DKA	diabetic ketoacidosis	PND	paroxysmal nocturnal dyspnoea
DM	diabetes mellitus		
DVT	deep vein thrombosis	PR	per rectum
FHx	family history	PUD	peptic ulcer disease
GB	gall bladder	PV	per vagina
GCA	giant cell arteritis	RA	rheumatoid arthritis
GI	gastrointestinal	SAH	subarachnoid haemorrhage
GORD	gastro-oesophageal reflux disease		
		SHx	social history
GTN	glyceryl trinitrate	SLE	systemic lupus erythematosus
GU	genitourinary		
HIV	human immunodeficiency virus	SOB	shortness of breath
		TB	tuberculosis
HRT	hormone replacement therapy	UTI	urinary tract infection
		VF	ventricular fibrillation
IBD	inflammatory bowel disease	VT	ventricular tachycardia
IBS	irritable bowel syndrome		

'Do you have tummy pain or discomfort?'

ΔΔ   *Inflammatory:* appendicitis, cholecystitis, pancreatitis, salpingitis, pyelonephritis, diverticulitis, inflammatory bowel disease.
Mechanical: intestinal obstruction, renal colic, biliary colic, ovarian torsion, testicular torsion.
Perforation: peptic ulcer, diverticulitis, appendix, GB, ruptured ectopic pregnancy, ruptured spleen or AAA.
Vascular: mesenteric infarction; AAA, sickle cell crisis.
Other: IBS, MI, DKA, basal pneumonia, porphyria.

T   Time of onset; speed of onset (seconds, minutes, hours, days). Progression over time, previous similar episodes.

I   Aggravating factors: e.g. food, breathing, movement, coughing. Relieving factors: e.g. lying still, sitting forward, analgesics, vomiting, bowel movement, micturition.

N   Main site of pain; unilateral/bilateral; *degree of localization*; radiation; has it moved? Character of pain (dull, sharp, stabbing, gnawing, colicky). Has the character of pain changed over time?
Constant or fluctuating in intensity (waxing and waning)?
Severity (out of 10, worst ever pain? cf. labour pains, toothache).

A   Vomiting, constipation, bloating (obstruction).
Dysuria, haematuria, frequency (renal colic, pyelonephritis, UTI).
Diarrhoea, blood/mucus PR, tenesmus (colitis, diverticulitis).
Haematemesis, melaena (gastric/duodenal ulcer).
Jaundice, pruritus, dark urine (obstructed common bile duct).
Lightheaded, feeling faint, collapse (ruptured ectopic/AAA).

PMHx   PUD, IBD, gallstones, IBS, GORD, PID; vascular disease, depression, anxiety, previous GI surgery or investigations, trauma.

DHx   Aspirin, NSAIDs, steroids, contraceptives/HRT, drug compliance.

FHx   IBD, PUD.

SHx   Alcohol, foreign travel, sexual partners, LMP, contraceptive use, life events and stresses.

'Has your appetite or weight changed recently?'

ΔΔ	Malignancy, chronic infection (TB, HIV, endocarditis), chronic disease (COPD, heart failure, liver failure, renal failure), malabsorption, thyrotoxicosis, Addison's disease, diabetes mellitus, anorexia nervosa, depression.
T	Duration; amount and rate of weight loss over 3, 6, 12 months.* Has weight loss plateaued or is it continuing?
I	Aggravating factors: stress, recent illness, eating alone. Relieving factors: eating with friends/family.
N	No desire to eat, vomiting, dysphagia or early satiety. Noticeable change in appearance, waist or clothes sizes decreasing. Objective evidence from clinic records of weight. Change in diet, intentional weight loss, weight loss accompanied by decreased food intake.
A	Amenorrhoea, negative body image (anorexia nervosa). Diarrhoea, steatorrhoea (malabsorption). Cough, dyspnoea, haemoptysis (TB, lung malignancy). Food intake maintained (thyrotoxicosis, diabetes). Low mood, anhedonism ↓ libido, poor sleep (depression). Dysphagia, altered bowel habit, anaemia, jaundice (GI malignancy). Fever, night sweats, malaise (chronic infection, lymphoma).
PMHx	Malignancy, chronic disease, GI or endocrine disease, rheumatic fever, prosthetic heart valve, depression.
DHx	Thyroxine, diuretics.
FHx	Diabetes mellitus, thyroid disease, coeliac disease, malignancy.
SHx	Alcohol intake, deliberate change in diet or exercise, smoking, drug abuse (cocaine, amphetamines), recent life stresses or bereavement, self-image, ethnic origin, travel history, sexual history.

---

* Weight loss of less than 3 kg in the previous 3 months is rarely of significance.

'Have you experienced any blackouts or funny turns?'

ΔΔ *Vasovagal syncope, cardiogenic syncope,* * *seizure*, postural hypotension, situational syncope (e.g. cough, micturition), carotid sinus hypersensitivity (CSH), vertebrobasilar insufficiency.

T Duration of problem; number and frequency of episodes, period of unconsciousness, speed of recovery.

I Aggravating factors: fear, intense emotion, prolonged standing (vasovagal†), standing up quickly (postural), sleep deprivation, alcohol excess or withdrawal, recreational drugs, flickering lights (seizure), exertion, no precipitant (cardiogenic), head movements (carotid sinus hypersensitivity, vertebrobasilar insufficiency).

Relieving factors: lying down/putting head down (vasovagal).

N Prodromal features: nausea, weakness, lightheadedness, pallor, sensations of heat, tinnitus, dimming of vision (vasovagal); aura,‡ abnormal focal movements (seizure), no warning (cardiac).

Loss of consciousness:§ incontinence, injury, tongue biting.

Eyewitness account: 'please describe exactly what happened', duration of attack, floppy or stiff, twitching or jerking, urinary or faecal incontinence (seizure), tongue biting (seizure), change in complexion, absent pulse.

After the attack: prolonged confusion or drowsiness (seizure), rapid complete recovery (cardiogenic).

A Palpitation, dyspnoea, chest pain (cardiogenic).

PMHx Epilepsy, ischaemic heart disease, valvular heart disease, arrhythmias, head injury, meningoencephalitis.

DHx Anticonvulsants (compliance), antiarrhythmic, antihypertensives.

FHx Epilepsy, ischaemic heart disease, hypertrophic cardiomyopathy.

SHx Recreational drugs, alcohol, sleep, foreign travel.

---

* Outflow obstruction, e.g. aortic stenosis; tachyarrhythmia, e.g. VT or VF; bradyarrhythmia, e.g. complete heart block.

† Vasovagal syncope is unlikely if attacks occur lying flat, e.g. in bed.

‡ Feelings of 'déjà vu' or 'jamais vu', flashing lights, strange noises, funny smells.

§ LOC is more likely to have occurred if the subject does not remember hitting the ground.

'Do you ever feel breathless or out of breath?'

ΔΔ   *Respiratory:* asthma, COPD, pneumonia, TB, pneumothorax, PE, lung malignancy, pulmonary fibrosis, LVF.
Other: metabolic acidosis, anaemia, shock, anxiety.

T   Occurs at rest or only on exertion, duration, speed of onset progression, pattern (persistent or episodic), worse at any particular time of day (see Fig. 5.1, p. 84).

I   Aggravating factors: pets, dust, etc. (asthma), exertion or lying supine (COPD, LVF, fibrosis, malignancy).
Relieving factors: inhalers (asthma/COPD), GTN spray (LVF, angina).

N   Severity (quantify exercise tolerance, ability to speak full sentences, frequency of inhaler use, cf. previous episodes).

A   Wheeze (asthma, COPD), calf pain/swelling (PE).
Pleuritic pain (PE, pneumonia, pneumothorax).
Anorexia, weight loss, haemoptysis (bronchial carcinoma, TB).
Fever, rigors, purulent sputum (pneumonia).
Dry, unproductive cough (fibrosis, LVF).
Chest pain, ankle swelling, nocturnal cough (LVF).
Pallor, lightheadedness, fatigue (anaemia).

PMHx   Respiratory/cardiac disease, DVT, GI bleeding, connective tissue disease or rheumatoid arthritis (fibrosis), previous admissions, previous assisted ventilation/home CPAP.

DHx   Inhalers, home nebulizers, home oxygen, oral steroids, diuretics, NSAIDs, methotrexate (pneumonitis), amiodarone (fibrosis).

FHx   Atopy, DVT/PE, TB.

SHx   Smoking history, occupation, asbestos exposure, travel/residence abroad, country of birth, pets, allergies.

'Have you had any pain or discomfort in your chest?'

ΔΔ	*Cardiac:* MI, angina, aortic dissection, pericarditis, massive PE. *Non-cardiac:* pleuritic, oesophageal, biliary, musculoskeletal.
T	Duration (< 20 min unlikely to be MI); sudden or more gradual onset; any previous similar episodes?
I	*Aggravating factors:* exercise, cold, emotion (angina), inspiration, coughing (pericarditis, pleuritic); local pressure (musculoskeletal); spicy food, alcohol, lying flat (oesophageal). *Relieving factors:* GTN, rest (angina); antacids (oesophageal); NSAIDs, sitting forward (pericarditis); nil (MI, aortic dissection).
N	Main site: retrosternal (angina, MI, dissection, GORD); lateralized (pericarditis, pleuritic, musculoskeletal). Radiation: arms, neck, jaw (MI, angina), interscapular (dissection). Character: tight, constricting, heavy, pressure (ischaemic), tearing (dissection), sharp, stabbing (pericarditis, pleuritic), hot, burning (GORD); similar to previous episodes of angina/MI? Severity (cf. normal anginal episodes; see p. 62).
A	Breathlessness, sweating, nausea, vomiting, angor animi (MI*). Haemoptysis, calf pain/swelling (PE). Focal neurological symptoms, haematuria (aortic dissection). Cough, sputum, breathlessness, shallow breathing (pleuritic).
PMHx	Previous MI; angina (frequency, exercise tolerance, response to GTN, attacks at rest); IHD risk factors (see p. 62); peripheral vascular disease, cerebrovascular disease DVT/PE, GORD, Marfan's syndrome.†
DHx	GTN, antiplatelets, antianginals, antihypertensives, statins, antacids, acid-lowering therapy.
FHx	MI (especially if age < 65), aortic dissection (hypertension).
SHx	Smoking (pack years), diet, exercise, alcohol.

---

* Factors increasing the likelihood of MI include age ≥ 65, past history of IHD, pressure-like character of pain, similarity of pain to previous MI, radiation of pain to *one* or *both* arms duration > 20 min.

† 25–50% of Marfan's syndrome patients die from aortic rupture or dissection.

'Have you lost track of time or become confused?'
'Can you tell me where you are and why you are here?'

ΔΔ   *Infection:* pneumonia, meningoencephalitis, septicaemia, hepatobiliary, diverticulitis, pyelonephritis, malaria.
Toxicity: alcohol (acute intoxication/withdrawal), recreational drugs (especially opiates), drug overdose.
Drugs: opiate analgesics, sedatives and antidepressants.
Vascular: stroke, MI, subdural haematoma, major GI bleed.
Metabolic: hypothermia, hypoxia, dehydration, hypothyroidism, hypo/hypernatraemia, hypo/hypercalcaemia, uraemia, hypo/hyperglycaemia, hepatic encephalopathy, depression.
Neurological: raised intracranial pressure, space-occupying lesion, head injury, dementia, post-ictal state, Wernicke–Korsakoff encephalopathy.

Explore all avenues for further information (friends, relatives, bystanders, GP, medical records, ambulance crew).

T   Acute or chronic, duration, rate of deterioration, previous episodes.

I   Aggravating factors: night-time, medications, fasting, exercise, alcohol, recreational drugs, overdose, sepsis, head injury.
Relieving factors: daylight, food, alcohol, drugs, antibiotics.

N   What is the patient's normal mental state? How much has this changed? Any evidence of forgetfulness or bizarre behaviour?

A   Fever, sweats, shivering, rigors (infection), hallucinations, restless or apathetic, headache, focal CNS signs (raised ICP, head injury, meningitis, intracranial bleed), cough, purulent sputum, dysuria, jaundice (hepatobiliary infection, hepatic encephalopathy)

PMHx   Dementia, recent falls/head injury/operations, CVA, depression, alcohol abuse, liver disease, deliberate self-harm, epilepsy.

DHx   See above. Any recent changes?

FHx   Epilepsy, diabetes.

SHx   Alcohol, recreational drugs, travel abroad, diet, social support.

'Have you noticed any change in your bowel habit?'
'Do you have to strain to open your bowels?'

ΔΔ   Intestinal obstruction, colorectal cancer, irritable bowel syndrome, low fibre/fluid intake, immobility (especially elderly), drug therapy, hypothyroidism, hypercalcaemia.

T   Acute or chronic? How long has constipation been a problem? Is it getting better or worse?

I   Aggravating factors: medications, menstruation, inactivity. Relieving factors: laxatives, exercise, dietary fibre.

N   What does the patient mean by constipation? (infrequent stools, small-volume stools, hard/firm stools, difficulty in defecation). Patient's normal bowel habit – has it changed recently? Frequency of bowel movements (number per week). Consistency, size, shape and colour of stools. Severity: how long spent straining at stool; impact on lifestyle.

A   Abdominal pain and distension, vomiting (obstruction). Anaemia, rectal bleeding, weight loss (colorectal cancer). Alternating bowel habit, abdominal pain, bloating (IBS).

PMHx   Hernias, previous abdominal surgery (adhesions), colorectal cancer, Crohn's disease, results of previous colonoscopy and/ or barium X-ray studies.

DHx   Opiates (including codeine), verapamil, anticholinergics, iron.

FHx   Colorectal cancer.

SHx   Diet, fluid intake, exercise.

'Have you noticed a change in your bowel habit?'
'Do you have to rush to empty your bowels? Are the stools loose?'

ΔΔ   *Acute* (< 10 days): infective gastroenteritis, drugs (e.g. antibiotics), food intolerance, food allergy, alcohol excess, ulcerative colitis.

Chronic/relapsing: IBS, IBD, drugs, laxatives, alcohol, malabsorption, infection, colorectal cancer, short bowel syndrome, autonomic neuropathy, thyrotoxicosis.

T   Speed of onset, progression, duration; intermittent or constant. Does diarrhoea alternate with constipation? (IBS).

I   Aggravating factors: adverse drug effect, alcohol abuse, specific foodstuffs, stressful events.

Relieving factors: opioids, drugs, intake restricted to water only (failure to resolve on starvation suggests a secretory diarrhoea).

N   What does the patient mean by diarrhoea (loose stools, watery stools, frequent stools, large volume of stool, urgency to defecate, incontinence)? How much stool is passed per day and how often?*

What is the normal bowel habit and has it changed in frequency or consistency? How often does diarrhoea occur? Does diarrhoea occur overnight? (suggests organic pathology). Is there abdominal pain with the diarrhoea? (absence of pain suggests malabsorption).

A   Blood (infective colitis, colorectal cancer, diverticulitis, IBD). Mucus, pus, slime (IBD, IBS, rectal tumour). Frequency and tenesmus (IBD, colitis, rectal cancer, IBS). Abdominal pain, weight loss (malignancy, malabsorption, IBD).

PMHx   Surgery/radiotherapy, previous endoscopies/barium X-rays.
DHx   Laxatives, antidiarrhoeal agents, antacids, antibiotics.
FHx   IBD, coeliac disease, colorectal cancer.
SHx   Travel abroad, contact with affected individuals, high-risk sexual behaviour (HIV), alcohol abuse, diet.

---

*   Large volumes, at infrequent intervals suggest small bowel disease; small volumes at frequent intervals suggest large bowel disease.

'Do you ever feel dizzy, lightheaded or unsteady?

ΔΔ   *Vertigo:** labyrinthine disorders (benign positional vertigo, Ménière's disease); vestibular nerve (acute labyrinthitis, acoustic neuroma); brain stem CVA.
Presyncope:† vasovagal, postural hypotension, anaemia, arrhythmia.
Loss of coordination:‡ cerebellar or brain stem dysfunction, CVA, alcohol abuse, multiple sclerosis, sensory ataxia, weakness.

T   Duration, time of day, acute or chronic, episodic or persistent. Relationship to posture/head movement.

I   Aggravating factors: head movement, motion (vertigo), alcohol (cerebellar), standing (vasovagal, postural hypotension, anaemia), poor light (sensory ataxia).
Relieving factors: lying down, eyes open or shut, sitting down.

N   Illusion of movement, loss of consciousness, familiar feelings prior to a simple faint (buzzing in ears, dimming of vision, etc.).

A   Nausea and vomiting (any cause of vertigo).
Hearing loss, tinnitus (labyrinthine or vestibular nerve disorder).
Cranial nerve palsies (acoustic neuroma, central lesion).
Loss of consciousness (any presyncopal cause; not vertigo).
Palpitations, chest pain, SOB, syncope (arrhythmia, anaemia).

PMHx   CVA, MS, recent head/facial trauma (vestibular nerve), previous faints, IHD, cardiac arrhythmias, DM.

DHx   Aminoglycosides, furosemide (frusemide).

SHx   Alcohol consumption.

---

* Vertigo: the illusion of movement (often but not always rotatory) of the patient or surroundings accompanied by a feeling of impaired balance.
† Presyncope: a feeling of lightheadedness as if about to faint.
‡ Loss of coordination: unsteadiness of gait with poor balance without any feeling of lightheadedness or vertigo (like being on a small boat).

'Do you have any difficulty in swallowing?'

ΔΔ *Mechanical:* oesophageal or gastric cancer, peptic stricture, extrinsic compression (e.g. bronchial cancer), pharyngeal pouch.
Non-mechanical: achalasia, myasthenia gravis, systemic sclerosis, bulbar or pseudobulbar palsy, Chagas' disease.

T Acute or chronic; intermittent or persistent; progressive.
I Difficulty mainly with solids (suggests mechanical obstruction).
Difficulty mainly with liquids (suggests neuromuscular problem).
N Painful (suggests disease with intact innervation, e.g. GORD).
Painless (suggests mucosal denervation, e.g. cancer).
What foods and/or liquids cause the problem?
What level does food stick in the oesophagus?
Is food regurgitated or does it eventually go down?
A Weight loss, anorexia, jaundice? (malignancy).
Choking or spluttering (impaired neuromuscular mechanisms).
Gurgling in the throat during eating (pharyngeal pouch).
Voice change (recurrent laryngeal nerve compression).
Nocturnal cough and breathlessness (gastric aspiration).

PMHx GORD, Barrett's oesophagus, HIV (candidiasis), radiotherapy.
DHx Long-term steroids (candidiasis).
FHx Oesophageal or gastric cancer.
SHx Smoking, alcohol, ethnic origin, residence in South America (Chagas' disease).

'Have you vomited any blood or brown fluid?'
'Have you passed any blood in your bowel motions or on the toilet paper?'
'Have you noticed any change in the colour of your bowel motions?'
'Have the bowel motions appeared black and tarry?'

ΔΔ   *Upper GI bleeding:* nosebleed, oesophagitis, peptic ulcer, Mallory–Weiss tear, varices, oesophageal or gastric tumour.
       Lower GI bleeding: colorectal tumours, diverticulitis, colitis (infective, ischaemic, antibiotic-associated, IBD), angiodysplasia, haemorrhoids, anal fissure, rectal prolapse.

T   Duration (days or weeks), intermittent or persistent, past episodes.
I   Alcoholic binging, NSAIDs and other drugs (see below).
N   Appearance of vomit/stools (bright red, clots, coffee-grounds).*
       How much blood passed? How many episodes?
       Have the stools changed in colour?†
A   Lightheadedness on standing? (significant volume loss).
       Prior indigestion or heartburn (peptic disease).
       Altered bowel habit ± weight loss, anorexia (colon cancer).
       Diarrhoea, abdominal pain ± fever (diverticulitis, colitis).
       Anal pain on defecation? (anal fissure or piles).

PMHx   Peptic ulcer, liver disease, colorectal tumour, IBD, diverticulitis, radiotherapy, peripheral vascular disease, previous investigations (barium studies, endoscopies).
DHx   Aspirin, NSAIDs, steroids, anticoagulants, clopidogrel, antibiotics.
FHx   Peptic ulcer, GI tumours, IBD.
SHx   Alcohol ingestion, travel abroad.

---

*   Bright red blood in vomit suggests pharyngeal or oesophageal bleeding; coffee-ground vomit suggests bleeding from the stomach or duodenum; profuse dark red vomit with clots suggests major upper GI haemorrhage. Retching without blood in the first vomit suggests oesophageal trauma (Mallory–Weiss syndrome).
†   Bright red blood on the stools or toilet paper usually arises from the anorectum; dark red blood mixed in with stool indicates a colonic lesion; black tarry motions (melaena) indicates upper GI bleeding.

'Have you had any headaches recently?

ΔΔ	Intracranial bleed (SAH), meningitis, encephalitis, trauma, tension headache, migraine, cluster headache, raised intracranial pressure (ICP), e.g. tumour, giant cell arteritis (GCA), otitis media, trigeminal neuralgia.
T	Speed of onset* (seconds, minutes, hours, days), frequency, time of onset (early morning suggests ↑ ICP) progression over time,† duration, prodromal symptoms, past episodes, recent change.
I	Aggravating factors: specific foodstuffs (cheese, chocolate, wine) or hunger (migraine); sexual intercourse (SAH, benign coital headache), stress (tension headache), bending, lying, straining (↑ ICP), bright lights or loud noises (migraine), chewing, trigeminal neuralgia.
	Relieving factors: simple analgesics, sitting up (↑ ICP), steroids (↑ ICP, GCA), relaxation (tension headache), lying still (migraine).
N	Site: unilateral/bilateral; ocular, temporal (GCA), occipital (SAH).
	Character: tight band, pressure (tension headache), dull, throbbing (migraine), explosive, 'thunderclap' (SAH).
	Severity: (out of 10, worst ever pain?, cf. toothache).
A	Neck stiffness, photophobia, ↓ consciousness (SAH, meningitis).
	Purpuric rash, fever (meningitis).
	Nausea, photophobia, phonophobia, malaise, aura‡ (migraine).
	Unilateral lacrimation, nasal congestion (cluster headache).
	Scalp tenderness and jaw claudication (arteritis).
	Loss of visual acuity with red eye and haloes (glaucoma).
	Morning vomiting, seizures, behavioural change (↑ ICP).
PMHx	Migraine, head injury, hypertension, depression/anxiety.
DHx	Nitrates, vasodilator therapy, daily analgesic use, OCP.
FHx	Migraine, Ménière's disease, SAH.
SHx	Alcohol abuse, stresses and difficulties, travel (malaria).

---

* Cerebral haemorrhage and SAH typically produce a severe headache of sudden onset.

† Short history with rapid progression suggests a more serious underlying problem.

‡ Typical aura includes visual scintillations or altered sensations especially paraesthesiae.

'Do you have difficulty getting around? Have you fallen recently?'

ΔΔ | *Predisposing factors:** impaired homeostasis, environmental factors (e.g. poor lighting, loose rugs), dementia, visual impairment, cerebrovascular disease, Parkinson's disease, arthritis of weight-bearing joints, drugs (see below).
Acute illness: infection (sepsis, pneumonia), stroke, fracture (neck of femur, vertebral), dehydration, MI, LVF, anaemia, renal failure, polymyalgia rheumatica, hypothermia, spinal cord compression.

T | Gradual or sudden deterioration, previous falls or episodes of immobility. When was the patient last able to go outdoors alone?

I | Time of day; medications (recent changes).

N | What is the patient's normal level of function? Is the patient able to get out of bed or a chair unaided? Generalized or local weakness. Movement limited by pain (fractures and arthritis).
Exact circumstances of falls (trip, slip, blackout or unsteadiness), injuries, witnesses, time spent on floor, loss of consciousness (p. 21).

A | Localized pain, bruising, swelling (fracture, soft tissue injury).
Fever, sweats, cough, sputum (pneumonia).
Chest pain, dyspnoea, orthopnoea, PND (MI, LVF).
Speech problems, focal weakness, tremor (CVA, Parkinson's disease).

PMHx | Previous falls, dementia, Parkinson's disease, cardiorespiratory disease, cerebrovascular disease, osteoarthritis, renal disorder, malignancy, recent trauma or head injury.

DHx | Benzodiazepines, phenothiazines, antidepressants, antihistamines, antihypertensives, diuretic, ACE inhibitors, sleeping tablets.

FHx | Stroke, hypertension, IHD, diabetes mellitus.

SHx | Social support, opportunities to get out, confidence, alcohol intake.

---

* Physiological changes in the ageing process include cerebral atrophy (cognitive impairment), cochlear degeneration (impaired hearing), dorsal column loss (sensory ataxia), anterior horn cell loss (muscle atrophy and weakness), lens opacification (impaired sight), impaired thermoregulation, impaired immune function, loss of bone density (low-impact fractures) and impaired renal medullary function (impaired urine concentration and drug elimination).

'Have you noticed any change in the colour of your skin or urine?'

ΔΔ	*Prehepatic:* Gilbert's syndrome, haemolysis (any cause).
	Hepatic: hepatitis (e.g. alcohol, viral, autoimmune, drugs); cirrhosis (any cause), malignancy (primary or secondary).
	Posthepatic: gallstones, pancreatic or cholangiocarcinoma.

T   Duration and speed of progression, painful or painless, previous episodes, intermittent or persistent, relapsing and remitting.

I   *Aggravating factors:* starvation (Gilbert's syndrome), drugs or alcohol.

Relieving factors: resolution of pain (gallstones or hepatitis).

N   Pale stools and dark urine (suggests posthepatic).

Absence of dark urine (suggests prehepatic).

Absence of systemic features (suggests Gilbert's syndrome).

A   Abdominal pain and anorexia (gallstones, hepatitis).

Weight loss and night sweats (malignancy).

Fever, breathlessness and tiredness (haemolysis).

Anxiety, depression, suicide risk factors (paracetamol overdose).

PMHx   Liver disease, pancreatitis, biliary surgery, previous jaundice, blood transfusion, depression, deliberate self-harm.

DHx   Antibiotics, paracetamol (overdose).

FHx   Jaundice (Gilbert's syndrome, epidemic infectious hepatitis).

SHx   Alcohol intake, travel abroad, high-risk sexual behaviour, intravenous drug abuse, skin tattoos, suspicious foods (shellfish).

'Do you have any pain or stiffness in your joints?'

ΔΔ   Osteoarthritis, rheumatoid arthritis, SLE, septic arthritis, trauma, gout, pseudogout, psoriatic arthropathy, reactive arthritis, ankylosing spondylitis, polymyalgia rheumatica.

T   Duration, mode of onset (acute or insidious), pattern (persistent, episodic, migratory or additive), progression over time.

I   *Aggravating factors:* pain and stiffness decrease on activity and increase on resting in inflammatory arthritis, cf. osteoarthritis. *Relieving factors:* rest (in OA), NSAIDs, steroids. Diurnal variation of pain or stiffness.

N   Which joints affected – monoarticular, oligoarticular, poly-articular, symmetrical or asymmetrical involvement? Presence/degree of pain, stiffness, swelling, immobility, weakness. *Severity:* how painful (disturbing sleep). *Limitation of activity:* activities of daily living/work.

A   *Systemic:* malaise, fever, sweats, myalgia, weight loss. *Skin:* rashes, photosensitivity (SLE), subcutaneous nodules (RA), tophi (gout), plaques and nail changes (psoriasis), alopecia (SLE), Raynaud's phenomenon (RA, SLE). *Eye:* dryness, redness, irritation, pain, ↓ acuity (Reiter's syndrome, RA, SLE). *Lung:* dyspnoea, cough, pleuritic pain (RA, SLE). *GI/GU:* diarrhoea, genital ulcers, discharge (reactive/Reiter's).

PMHx   OA, RA, SLE, gout, psoriasis, IBD, recent trauma/injury, recurrent miscarriages/thromboses, recent throat, GI or GU infection.

DHx   Current and previous treatments (disease-modifying anti-rheumatic drugs, NSAIDs, steroids), diuretics.

FHx   Rheumatoid arthritis, SLE, ankylosing spondylitis, IBD, psoriasis, gout.

SHx   Impact of symptoms on daily activities, employment, social functioning, sexual intercourse, physical sports, hobbies, travel abroad.

'Have you felt sick or squeamish?'
'When did you last vomit?'

ΔΔ	*GI:* Gastroenteritis, peptic ulcer, gastric outlet obstruction, bowel obstruction, ileus, cholecystitis, hepatitis, pancreatitis. *CNS:* ↑ ICP, migraine, Ménière's, brainstem disease. *Metabolic:* ↑ Ca, uraemia, ↓ Na, DKA, Addison's disease. *Other:* Drugs, pregnancy, alcohol, severe pain, bulimia, sepsis, disseminated malignancy.
T	Duration, time of day/month, relationship to food. Chronic or acute, episodic or persistent.
I	Aggravating factors: food, motion, alcohol. Relieving factors: lying still, antiemetics.
N	Number of vomits, projectile (pyloric stenosis), bloodstained, bile-stained, feculent (gastrocolic fistula), absence of nausea (↑ ICP), colour, quantity, smell of vomit.
A	Abdominal pain, distension, constipation (bowel obstruction, ileus). Diarrhoea (infective gastroenteritis, antibiotics). Fever, sweats, rigors (cholecystitis, sepsis). Headache ± aura (migraine, ↑ ICP). Vertigo, hearing loss, tinnitus (Ménière's disease). Weight loss, anorexia, cachexia (malignancy). Jaundice (hepatitis, gallstones, malignancy). Polyuria (DKA or ↑ Ca). Delayed menstrual period (pregnancy).
PMHx	See ΔΔ, abdominal surgery, hernias, renal failure, DM, hyperparathyroidism, psychiatric history.
DHx	Digoxin, opiates, antibiotics, antidepressants.
FHx	Migraine, peptic ulcer.
SHx	Alcohol or drug abuse, LMP, suspicious foodstuffs, foreign travel.

Breast lump Ask about duration of lump, previous lumps/mammography, change in size over time and with menstrual cycle and presence of nipple discharge or pain as well as participation in screening programmes. Benign causes include cysts, fibroadenomas, periductal mastitis and localized fibroadenosis. Risk factors for breast carcinoma include ↑ age, previous breast cancer, FHx, nulliparity, early menarche, late menopause, first pregnancy > 30 years old, HRT.

Cough and sputum A dry, non-productive cough is typical of pulmonary fibrosis, ACE-inhibitor therapy and the early stages of pneumonia. In later stages of pneumonia a cough productive of purulent/rusty brown sputum is usual. Chronic productive cough is a feature of COPD and bronchiectasis. Cough tends to be more troublesome at night in asthma, pulmonary oedema and postnasal drip and more troublesome in the morning in COPD and bronchiectasis. Cough may lack its normal explosive character when a vocal cord is paralysed ('bovine' cough). See Table 5.2 (p. 84) for interpretation of sputum.

Deafness Common with advancing age; minor degrees are often overlooked. It may occur with *tinnitus* (buzzing or ringing in the ears) and *vertigo* (unsteadiness with a feeling of movement) – typical of inner ear disease. Conductive deafness is due to middle ear disease and sensorineural deafness is due to VIII nerve disorders.

Depression The cardinal feature is *anhedonism* (inability to feel pleasure and interest in life); ask what patients enjoys doing, what previously interested them and if it still does. Other features include reduced appetite and libido, weight loss, sleep disturbance with early morning waking, *psychomotor retardation* (slowness of movement and thought processes), unwarranted or excessive pessimism and feelings of guilt and worthlessness. Ask about suicidal feelings: 'When did you last feel life was not worth the effort?'; if present, ask about the details of the patient's plans for suicide and about any previous attempts.

Dysuria   Discomfort on passing urine due to lower urinary tract infection. Typically burning in nature and accompanied by *urgency* (sudden strong need to pass urine), *strangury* (unremitting desire to urinate) and ↑ urinary frequency. Other causes include urethritis (e.g. gonorrhoea), prostatitis and lower urinary tract stones or tumours.

Fatigue   Excessive tiredness associated with loss of drive; it is a common, non-specific feature of significant illness. Tiredness on exertion relieved by rest suggests IHD. When tiredness is the principal symptom, it is typically more marked on resting than exertion and is associated with a change in the pattern of sleep with features suggesting depression ± anxiety.

Flatulence   Belched wind has often been swallowed (*aerophagy*) without the patient's awareness. Belching itself is rarely of significance but may be a feature of anxiety and commonly accompanies upper abdominal pain or discomfort. Excessive flatus is particularly troublesome in carbohydrate malabsorption, e.g. lactase deficiency.

Haematuria   Presence of blood in urine: macroscopic when visible to the naked eye, microscopic when evident only on urine dipstick examination. It may be due to renal/ureteric stones when accompanied by severe loin pain, or to lower urinary tract infection especially if associated with dysuria and frequency. Painless haematuria is a common presenting feature of bladder tumours.

Haemoptysis   Volume may range from blood-staining of sputum to massive haemorrhage (e.g. bronchiectasis, tumour and aspergilloma). Take care to distinguish from heamatemesis. Recurrent haemoptysis, however modest, is more often clinically significant than a single episode and suggests the presence of bronchial carcinoma. The association of haemoptysis with pleuritic pain and breathlessness suggests pulmonary embolism – ask about calf symptoms and risk factors for DVT.

Heartburn   A retrosternal, burning discomfort; when it is the predominant symptom, it invariably indicates gastro-oesophageal reflux disease (GORD). Typically, it is induced by meals, bending down or lying on the left side and is common during pregnancy or following weight gain (due to ↑ intra-abdominal pressure).

Insomnia   Usually psychological in origin (ask patients what goes through their mind when lying awake) but exclude physical causes, e.g. thyrotoxicosis, nocturia, night sweats, breathlessness. Depression typically produces early morning waking. Ask about duration of problem, pattern of sleep disturbance, current stresses, alcohol intake, caffeine consumption and use of hypnotics.

Intermittent claudication   Cramping pain in calf muscles precipitated by walking and relieved by rest, usually due to disease of the superficial femoral artery. More proximal narrowing may produce exertional pain in the buttock. Ask about its severity (walking distance) and the presence of night pain and rest pain (indicating critical ischaemia). Consider alternative or additional diagnoses – anaemia, beta-blockade therapy and spinal claudication due to lumbar canal stenosis.

Menstrual disorders   *Dysmenorrhoea* (painful menstruation), *menorrhagia* (excessively heavy bleeding during periods), *amenorrhoea* (absence of periods) and *polymenorrhoea* (increased frequency of periods). *Postmenopausal bleeding* suggests endometrial carcinoma. Amenorrhoea commonly results from severe weight loss and major illness; it may be the presenting symptom of anorexia nervosa or pregnancy.

Oedema   Tissue swelling due to interstitial fluid caused by ↑ venous hydrostatic pressure (e.g. heart failure, DVT), ↓ capillary oncotic pressure from ↓ serum albumin (e.g. cirrhosis, nephrotic syndrome, protein-losing enteropathy) or lymphatic obstruction (e.g. malignant infiltration). Ask about drug therapy (calcium-channel blockers), duration, progression and associated symptoms, e.g. breathlessness.

Oliguria   Passing smaller volume of urine than normal (< 700 mL/day). Usually due to dehydration or acute renal failure. *Anuria* (complete absence of urine production) indicates urinary tract obstruction.

Painful mouth   Soreness of the lips, *cheilosis*, tongue, *glossitis*, or buccal mucosa, *stomatitis*, may be associated with iron, folate or vitamin B_{12} deficiency, dermatological disorders, chemotherapy and infection. Aphthous ulcers are common in gluten enteropathy and IBD.

Palpitation   Awareness of the heart beat may be due to cardiac arrhythmias but more commonly reflects anxiety or premature beats. Ask the patient whether the heart beat is fast or slow; regular or irregular; ask the patient to illustrate by tapping a finger on the chest. Ask about frequency of episodes, associated symptoms particularly dizziness, syncope and chest pain, possible precipitants (e.g. caffeine, alcohol, exertion) and a past history of cardiac or thyroid disease.

Paraesthesiae   Tingling or numbness due to involvement of sensory pathways at any site between the peripheral nerve and the parietal cortex.

Pneumaturia   Passage of air bubbles during urination because of a colovesical fistula (often diverticular abscess or colonic/bladder cancer).

Polyuria   Passing more urine than usual, irrespective of frequency. Causes include diabetes mellitus, diabetes insipidus, hypercalcaemia, chronic renal failure and *psychogenic polydipsia* (excessive drinking).

Prostatism   Obstruction to urine flow produces a poor urinary stream, *hesitancy* (difficulty in initiating micturition), and urinary dribbling after micturition, as well as urinary frequency and *nocturia* (passing urine during the night) due to incomplete bladder emptying. Causes include benign prostatic hypertrophy, prostatic carcinoma and urethral stricture.

Pruritus   Often due to skin disorders, e.g. eczema, scabies, urticaria. Ask about allergies, rashes, drug therapy, previous skin disorders and any close contacts with similar problems. Generalized itching is caused by systemic disorders (e.g. biliary tract obstruction, chronic renal failure, lymphoma, iron deficiency).

Sexual dysfunction   Men may present with *impotence* (inability to achieve or sustain erections), *premature ejaculation* or loss of libido. Women may present with loss of libido, inability to orgasm, *dyspareunia* (pain during or after intercourse) or *vaginismus* (vaginal spasm on attempted intercourse). Most sexual dysfunction has a psychological basis; physical causes include peripheral vascular disease and autonomic neuropathy (especially diabetes).

Strangury   Painful sensation of an unremitting desire to pass urine often due to bladder neck infection or obstruction.

Stridor   A *'crowing' sound* during breathing not unlike wheeze but differs in being more obvious during inspiration rather than expiration. It is often worse after coughing and indicates obstruction of the large airways (larynx or trachea). Its presence demands urgent assessment to exclude bronchial carcinoma and vocal cord paralysis.

Tenesmus   A feeling of incomplete rectal evacuation with a persistent desire to defecate; common in colitis, rectal carcinoma, rectal prolapse and irritable bowel syndrome.

Urinary incontinence   *Stress incontinence* (involuntary urination during coughing or laughing) is usually due to weakness of the pelvic floor muscles and often follows a difficult childbirth. *Urge incontinence* (inability to delay micturition following the call to void) is common in bladder infections but is also typical following stroke. Incontinence may result from the inability to access a toilet quickly, and reduced mobility is an important factor in the frail elderly subject.

Vaginal discharge   Presence of a vaginal discharge usually suggests infection. Ask about its colour and smell, itching/burning, presence of blood-staining and/or abdominal pain. Ask about the sexual history, change in sexual partner and any urinary symptoms or discharge that the partner may have experienced. It requires microbiological investigation.

Visual impairment   May comprise *photophobia* (intolerance of light), *photopsia* (seeing flashes and zig-zags of light), *diplopia* (double vision), *amblyopia* (blurred vision), loss of part of the field of vision of one eye (*scotoma*), loss of half of the field of vision of both eyes (*hemianopia*) or loss of one-quarter of the field of vision of both eyes (*quadrantanopia*). Ask about '*positive symptoms*' such as seeing haloes (*glaucoma*) and about '*negative symptoms*' such as loss of vision. Episodes of diplopia and blurred vision are common in multiple sclerosis. Transient diplopia is a typical presenting feature of myasthenia gravis. A transient visual disorder may be the prelude to a migrainous headache.

Water brash   Reflex hypersalivation often described as the mouth filling with tasteless fluid (cf. acid reflux with a sour taste in the mouth); it is an uncommon but characteristic feature of peptic ulcer disease.

Weakness   Muscle weakness arises from disorders of the upper or lower motor neurone, myoneural junction or muscles. It may be proximal, distal or global, symmetrical or asymmetrical in distribution. Check that the problem really is one of weakness rather than incoordination.

Wheeze   Musical polyphonic sounds (*rhonchi*) during breathing, more conspicuous during expiration. It is caused by obstruction of the small airways, e.g. asthma, and is often accompanied by breathlessness (*dyspnoea*). Ask about precipitants, e.g. exercise, dust, smoke, pets.

General examination

Relating the physical examination to the history

A detailed clinical history is usually more helpful in making the correct diagnosis than is the physical examination. The history should suggest a differential diagnosis and help you to focus your physical examination.

General principles of the physical examination

- Before you examine the patient, screen the bed or couch as appropriate to ensure privacy.
- Adjust the back rest; breathless patients are more breathless lying flat.
- Ensure good illumination; adequately expose the area to be examined but avoid embarrassing or chilling the patient.
- Make sure that the patient is warm; shivering causes muscle sounds which interfere with auscultation, and palpation with cold hands causes the abdominal muscles to contract, impairing the examination.
- Carry out your examination from the patient's right side if you are right-handed and from the left side if you are left-handed.
- Handle any painful area as gently as possible.
- Avoid exhausting the patient from prolonged examination, especially the sick, frail or elderly. If appropriate, complete the examination in several visits.
- Ask the medical or nursing staff for advice about chaperoning. Male students should be chaperoned when examining young females.
- Record your examination findings systematically. Use diagrams to define the site and extent of physical findings such as swellings or the effects of trauma.
- Identify the patient's active problems and differential diagnoses.
- Consider a management plan, including the further investigations necessary to establish the diagnosis and an outline of the treatment.

The setting

Observe the patient's immediate environment for clues (Fig. 3.1).

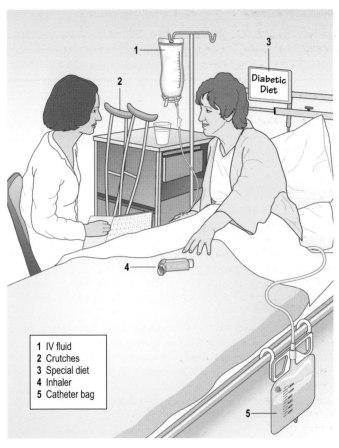

1 IV fluid
2 Crutches
3 Special diet
4 Inhaler
5 Catheter bag

Fig. 3.1 The setting.

Abnormal colours

Anaemia is best appreciated from the colour of the conjunctivae, nail beds and skin creases. Cyanosis, a deep red or bluish discoloration of the skin and mucous membranes, is caused by deoxygenated haemoglobin (>40 g/L), methaemoglobin (>15 g/L) or sulphaemoglobin (>5 g/L) (p. 86). Jaundice is best seen in the sclera and underneath the tongue; it can easily be missed in artificial light. Increased skin pigmentation is a feature of Addisonian adrenal failure, chronic liver disease and haemochromatosis; decreased skin pigmentation is seen in vitiligo, hypopituitarism, albinism and phenylketonuria.

Abnormal sounds

A hoarse, gruff voice may indicate severe hypothyroidism due to myxoedematous thickening of the vocal cords. *Stridor*, an inspiratory, crowing sound, suggests obstruction of the major airway (larynx, trachea or main bronchi). Hoarseness and difficulty phonating vowels suggest vocal cord paralysis due to recurrent laryngeal nerve palsy.

Abnormal odours

Halitosis, a malodorous breath, suggests gingivitis, poor dental hygiene or bronchiectasis. Foul-smelling, feculent belching may suggest a gastrocolic fistula. The sweet smell of acetone in the breath (cf. nail varnish remover) is typical of severe diabetic ketoacidosis; though obvious to some individuals, not all are able to detect it. A sickly-sweet smell of the breath, *fetor hepaticus*, occurs in liver failure.

Demeanour

The patient's demeanour, attitude and mood may be apparent from observation and analysis of the posture, gait, dress, mannerisms and behaviour. Both the verbal and non-verbal communication ('body language') give important complementary information.

Nutrition and hydration

Nutritional status is readily assessed by measuring the BMI and/or waist circumference (Table 3.1). Hydration is assessed by gently pinching the skin of the chest wall; the skin becomes lax and inelastic in pure water depletion.

3.1 Classification of obesity by BMI*, waist circumference (WC)# and associated disease risk±				
Status	BMI (kg/m²)	Obesity class	Normal WC (cm)	Abnormal WC (cm)
			♂ ≤ 102 ♀ ≤ 88	♂ > 102 ♀ > 88
Underweight	≤ 18.5			
Normal	18.5–24.9			
Overweight	25.0–29.9		↑	↑↑
Obesity	30.0–34.9	I	↑↑	↑↑↑
	35.0–39.9	II	↑↑↑	↑↑↑
Morbid obesity	≥ 40.0	III	↑↑↑↑	↑↑↑↑

* Body mass index (BMI) = weight (kg)/height (m)²
\# Waist circumference is less useful if the BMI > 35
± Increased waist circumference is a marker for an increased risk of type 2 diabetes mellitus, hypertension and cardiovascular disease even in persons of normal weight.

After the initial general inspection of the patient, the specific physical examination begins with inspection of the hands. For example, much can be learned about the patient from the appearance of the nails: well-groomed, bitten, ingrained with dirt or tobacco.

- **Skin:** *telangiectases* in cirrhosis of the liver or systemic sclerosis; an orange-yellow discoloration of the palms, *carotenaemia*, is typical in vegetarianism (also anorexia and hypothyroidism).
- **Subcutaneous tissue:** *rheumatoid nodules* around joints suggest rheumatoid arthritis. If nodules contain white spots, *tophi*, think of gout; if nodules are yellowish and attached to tendons, *xanthomata*, think of hypercholesterolaemia.
- **Nails:** *splinter haemorrhages* suggest infective endocarditis and nail 'spooning' (*koilonychia*) iron deficiency. Psoriasis may result in *nail pitting* and *onycholysis* (premature separation of the distal nail from the nail bed).
- **Muscles:** diffuse wasting and fasciculation of the small muscles of the hand suggest denervation, e.g. motor neurone disease.
- **Joints:** proximal interphalangeal joint disease suggests rheumatoid arthritis and distal interphalangeal joint disease (*Heberden's nodes*), primary generalized osteoarthritis.

Finger clubbing

- Inspect the nails noting the convexity of the nail.
- Look for disappearance of the nail bed angle.
- Look for fluctuation: rest the patient's finger on the pulp of your thumbs; palpate the base of the nail bed with both forefingers, pressing first with one finger and then the other. Fluctuation gives a characteristic floating sensation between the fingers (Fig. 3.2).

Clubbing, a bulbous swelling of the terminal phalanges of fingers and toes, is best characterized by increased nail bed fluctuation, increased convexity of the nail and loss of the hyponychial angle at the nail base (Fig. 3.3). Clubbing is occasionally congenital but its development usually indicates serious disease of the lungs, heart, liver or gut (Table 3.2).

3.2	Causes of finger clubbing
Respiratory	Bronchial carcinoma
	Bronchiectasis
	Empyema
	Lung abscess
	Fibrosing alveolitis
Cardiovascular	Cyanotic congenital heart disease
	Bacterial endocarditis
Alimentary	Hepatic cirrhosis
	Ulcerative colitis
	Crohn's disease
	Coeliac disease
Congenital	Familial clubbing

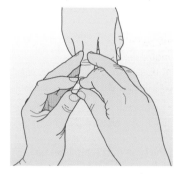

Fig. 3.2   Testing for fluctuation of the nail bed.

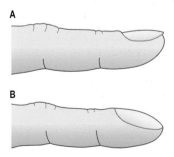

Fig. 3.3   Inspecting the nail bed angle.
Note the difference between (A) normal and (B) clubbing, with loss of nail bed angle and increased curvature of the nail.

Face

Facial appearances and expressions may be pathognomonic (Table 3.3).

Mouth

Examination of the mouth comprises inspection of the lips, tongue, teeth, gums, tonsils, palate, mucosa of the cheeks, salivary glands, floor of the mouth and the oropharynx.

- **Tongue:** cyanosis of the tongue is a good guide to central cyanosis (p. 86). Diffuse atrophy of the filiform papillae results in a smooth, clean-looking tongue in iron, folate or vitamin B_{12} deficiency. Carcinoma should be considered in the differential diagnosis of any chronic ulcer in or around the mouth. Excessive furring is of little diagnostic significance despite the patient's concern.
- **Teeth:** caries often results in loose teeth due to periodontitis; chronic gingivitis produces gum recession and is a major cause of dental losses. Gum hypertrophy can be a feature of phenytoin therapy or monocytic leukaemia. These disorders not only produce local symptoms but are important portals of bacterial entry causing endocarditis.
- **Tonsils:** reaching maximum size between the ages of 8 and 12 years, the tonsils then involute in adulthood.
- **Oropharynx:** pus from infection in the nose may sometimes be visible tracking down the back of the throat.
- **Parotid glands:** bilateral swelling of the parotids suggests chronic alcohol abuse (alcoholic sialoadenosis), mumps, Sjögren's syndrome or sarcoidosis (Heerfordt's syndrome). Unilateral swelling suggests parotitis, duct obstruction or tumour (pleomorphic adenoma).

Eyes (Table 3.4)

Examination of the eyes includes elements of both the general examination and specific examination for ophthalmological disorders and CNS disorders. It should also include ophthalmoscopy (p. 56).

3.3 Characteristic facies and their features, including facial expression	
Disorder	**Appearance**
Acromegaly	Coarsening with enlarged features, e.g. nose, lips, orbital ridges and jaw (prognathism)
Hypothyroidism	Malar flush, thickening with loss of the lateral third of the eyebrows
Hyperthyroidism	Startled appearance with lid retraction
Cushing's disease	'Moon-face', plethoric complexion and buffalo hump over lower cervical–upper thoracic spine
Parkinsonism	Expressionless facies and drooling mouth
Myasthenia gravis	Expressionless facies with bilateral ptosis
Myotonia dystrophica	Frontal baldness and bilateral ptosis
Superior vena caval (SVC) obstruction	Plethoric, oedematous face and neck, chemosis of the conjunctivae and prominent veins and venules
Malar flush	Dusky redness of cheeks seen in low cardiac output, e.g. mitral stenosis; also seen in myxoedema
Systemic lupus erythematosus	Rash over nose and cheeks – 'butterfly rash'
Progressive systemic sclerosis	Taut skin around the mouth with 'beaking' of the nose

3.4 Signs of systemic disorders affecting the eyes	
Colour of sclera	**Disorder**
Blue	Chronic iron deficiency
	Osteogenesis imperfecta
Yellow	Jaundice *but* not carotenaemia
Red	Scleritis in vasculitic disorders and rheumatoid disease
Black	Scleromalacia in rheumatoid disease

The neck should be inspected for any changes in the skin, scars, swellings and arterial and venous pulsation. Remember that the thyroid gland moves up on swallowing because it is enveloped by the pretracheal fascia, which is attached to the larynx.

- Examine the patient from behind with the patient sitting up.
- Palpate for cervical lymphadenopathy by positioning yourself behind the patient and systematically feeling and comparing the deep and superficial lymphatic chains on either side of the neck (p. 87).
- Examine for scalene lymph nodes: with the patient's neck slightly flexed and tilted towards the side being examined, insert the finger tip behind the sternocleidomastoid and the clavicle and feel deeply down onto the first rib, warning the patient of possible discomfort.
- Check the position of the trachea and its centrality (p. 90).
- Palpate the thyroid gland (Fig. 3.4) and define the characteristics of any goitre or mass. Ask the patient to swallow a sip of water to assess the movement on swallowing of any mass or goitre found.
- Auscultate for bruits over the thyroid gland and the carotid and subclavian arteries.
- Examine the internal and external jugular veins (p. 68).
- Assess neck movements and the cervical spine (p. 164).
- Assess the thyroid status of the patient, especially if a goitre is present (Table 3.5).

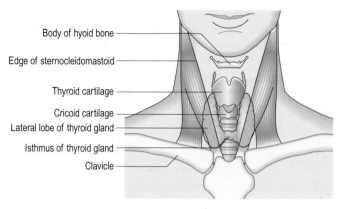

Body of hyoid bone

Edge of sternocleidomastoid

Thyroid cartilage

Cricoid cartilage

Lateral lobe of thyroid gland

Isthmus of thyroid gland

Clavicle

Fig. 3.4 Surface anatomy of the thyroid gland.

3.5 Assessment of thyroid status	
General inspection	Thin, anxious, sweaty, flushed, restless (hyper-) Overweight, thin dry hair, croaky voice (hypo-)
Face	Proptosis, exophthalmos, lid retraction/lag (hyper-) Coarse features, periorbital skin oedema (hypo-) Loss of hair in lateral third of eyebrows (hypo-) Malar flush (hypo-)
Hands	Hot sweaty palms, palmar erythema (hyper-) Cold, dry hands (hypo-)
Radial pulse	Tachycardia and bounding pulse, atrial fibrillation (hyper-) Bradycardia (hypo-)
Proximal muscle weakness of pectoral and pelvic girdle (hyper-) Supinator and ankle jerks for delayed relaxation (hypo-)	

Masses and skin lesions should be examined methodically to define the anatomical and pathological features, establish a diagnosis and plan the appropriate investigations.

Masses (SPASECTIT)

- **S**ize (measured with a tape) and shape: record using a diagram.
- **P**osition and relationships to adjacent structures: define accurately.
- **A**ttachments to skin and deeper structures: note its mobility or its fixation to neighbouring structures.
- **S**urface characteristics: note if smooth, lobulated or regular.
- **E**dge characteristics: note if sharp, blunt, well defined or diffuse.
- **C**onsistency: note if uniform, hard, rubbery, soft or fluctuant.
- **T**hrills or pulsations: vascular bruit? cough impulse? e.g. hernia.
- **I**nflammation: note presence of redness, heat, pain and tenderness.
- **T**ransillumination: use a pen-torch to assess if solid or cystic.

Skin lesions

- Examine the entire skin surface of the patient.
- Don't forget to examine the nails, mucous membranes (including the eyes and mouth), scalp, axillae, buttocks and perineum.
- Note the size, shape, colour, position and distribution of lesions.
- Define lesions using the appropriate descriptive terms (Tables 3.6 and 3.7).
- Use a magnifying glass (loop) as necessary.
- Record your findings using diagrams.

3.6 Dermatological glossary

Macule	A small circumscribed discoloration of the skin, such as a freckle
Papule	A palpable lesion raised above the surrounding surface of the skin
Vesicle (blister)	A lesion consisting of liquid within the epidermis or dermis
Bulla	A larger variety of vesicle
Pustule	A purulent vesicle
Erythema	Describes reddening of the skin

3.7 Common skin disorders

- **Eczema:** typically associated with allergic disorders in atopic subjects. Eczema is characterized by scaling or desquamation, due to abnormal maturation of the skin; areas commonly involved include the flexor surfaces of the arms and legs
- **Urticaria:** raised pale areas of skin due to interstitial fluid surrounded by erythema, is an allergic response characterized by capillary dilatation induced by an axon reflex
- **Psoriasis:** characterized by well-defined erythematous plaques with silvery scale which are usually found on the extensor surfaces and the scalp
- **Seborrhoeic keratosis:** usually appears as small, fleshy, yellow-brown papules on the trunk. They are due to basal cell papillomas and unrelated to the sebaceous glands. Their numbers increase markedly with age and are of no clinical significance
- **Cutaneous striae:** linear markings seen on the breasts, thighs and abdomen; those of recent origin are pink while older striae are whitish. They are due to stretching of the skin associated with rapid weight gain due to obesity, ascites or pregnancy. In Cushing's syndrome, purple striae appear over the pectoral regions and upper arms, the lower abdomen and upper thighs
- **Erythema nodosum:** characterized by painful, reddish-brown lumps on the shins, due to a hypersensitivity reaction to various drugs, allergens or infections, including sarcoidosis and primary tuberculosis
- **Skin tumours:** may be benign or malignant, primary or secondary. Basal cell carcinomas (rodent ulcers) are the commonest skin cancers and are common in the elderly, especially on the face. They rarely metastasize though they are locally invasive. In contrast, squamous cell carcinoma (*epithelioma*) is a rapidly growing tumour which spreads to adjacent tissues and lymph nodes at an early stage. *Melanomas* (*melanocytic naevi*) are benign moles; malignant transformation is rare but is suggested by enlargement, local itch, ulceration, colour change or the development of metastases
- **Purpura:** spontaneous cutaneous haemorrhages varying in size from tiny spots which *do not* blanch on pressure (*petechiae*) to large bruises (*ecchymoses*). Purpura results from increased capillary fragility or from thrombocytopenia

- Ask the patient if she would like a chaperone to be present.
- Ask the patient if she has noticed any breast lumps.
- Ask the patient to lie comfortably and to relax on the bed with her hands on her hips and her head on one pillow.
- Inspect the nipples, areolas and breasts: look for nipple inversion and discharge, asymmetry and skin changes around the nipples such as dimpling like the skin of an orange.
- Repeat the inspection (Fig. 3.5) as the patient presses her hands against her hips (contracting the pectoral muscles), with her hands raised above her head (stretching the pectoral muscles) and sitting forward with the breasts dependent.
- Ask the patient to place her hands behind her head: palpate each breast in turn by compressing the breast tissue against the chest wall using the palmar surface of the fingers held flat on the surface of the breast.
- Palpate the apex of the axilla and the chest wall for lymphadenopathy using the finger tips of either hand (Fig. 3.6).
- Record the characteristics of any lumps: size, position, attachments, mobility, surface, edge, consistency, signs of inflammation (tenderness, warmth and redness) and the date of the patient's last menstrual period.

Breast examination is best integrated into the physical examination immediately after the examination of the heart. The breast is a common site of carcinoma in women of all ages; any female in whom carcinoma is suspected should have the breasts examined carefully; any breast lump should be assessed as potentially malignant.

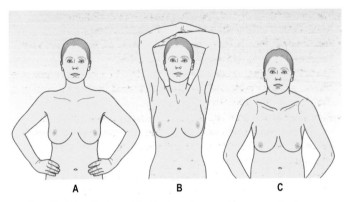

Fig. 3.5 Positions for inspecting the breast.
(A) Hands pressed into hips. (B) Hands above head. (C) Leaning forward.

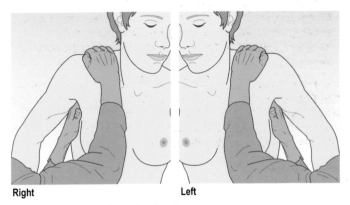

Right   Left

Fig. 3.6 Palpation of the axillary lymph nodes.

- If appropriate, dilate the pupils using tropicamide 1% eye drops; alternatively, perform the examination in a darkened room.
- Remove both the patient's and the examiner's spectacles and make the appropriate correction for refractive errors.
- Hold the ophthalmoscope with a forefinger on the lens adjustment wheel.
- Use your right eye to look at the patient's right eye and your left eye to look at the patient's left eye (Fig. 3.7).
- Ask the patient to focus on a specific distant object, to breathe normally and to blink as necessary.
- Set the ophthalmoscope lens to zero, shine the light beam into the pupil from a distance of about 15 cm and look for the red reflex (Table 3.8).
- Examine the fundus by moving the ophthalmoscope closer to the patient (normally 3–4 cm from the patient's eyeball) and adjusting the focus as necessary until the retinal vessels look sharp and clear.
- Locate the optic disc by following the course of an artery or a vein centrally and notice the sharpness of the edge of the optic disc, its colour and the depth of the optic cup (Fig. 3.8).
- Inspect the arteries and veins, noting their width and colour, the light reflex along the centre of the arterioles and the appearance at arteriovenous crossings. Then follow the vessels out into the peripheral aspects of the fundus.
- Study the appearance of the fundus systematically by radiating from the disc to the periphery, right round in a clockwise or anticlockwise manner. Note the position of haemorrhages, exudates or other abnormality.
- Examine the macula and its surroundings by asking the patient to look directly into the light; if necessary narrow the light beam.
- Record the ophthalmological findings diagrammatically.

3.8 Red reflex

- The red reflex is the initial assessment of the visibility of the retina
- In the normal reflex the pupil will shine red when visualized through the ophthalmoscope
- Opacification of the cornea, lens or vitreous humour can obscure the reflex completely (dense widespread). However, smaller opacities will be outlined black against the glow of the red reflex

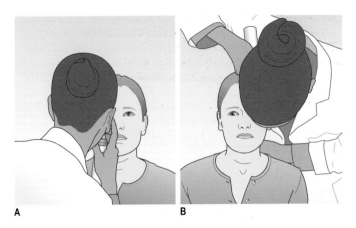

Fig. 3.7   Ophthalmoscopic technique.
(A) Conventional examination of patient's right eye using your own right eye.
(B) Examination from above if unable to use left eye to examine patient's left eye.

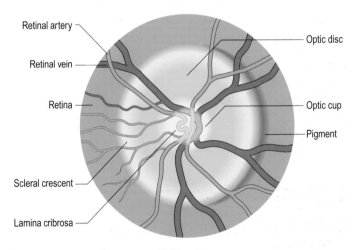

Fig. 3.8   The optic disc anatomy (right eye).

- Examine the external ear: look at the pinna and external meatus for evidence of inflammation, gouty tophi or any other abnormality.
- Hold the auriscope like a pen: insert the speculum of the auriscope into the meatus while gently retracting the pinna of the ear upwards and backwards, straightening the external canal to facilitate entry.
- Identify the tympanic membrane: look for the cone of reflected light from the handle of the malleus denoting a healthy eardrum (Fig. 3.9). Note any redness, bulging or perforation of the eardrum.

Auriscopic examination is indicated if there is earache or deafness. The normal tympanic membrane is pearly grey but in acute otitis media, it will be red and bulging and with no light reflex (Table 3.9).

Testing the hearing is described on page 132.

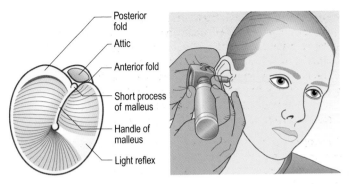

Posterior fold
Attic
Anterior fold
Short process of malleus
Handle of malleus
Light reflex

Fig. 3.9   Position for auriscopic examination and tympanic membrane anatomy.

3.9	Common abnormalities on auriscopy
Aetiology	**Clinical findings**
Otitis externa	Erythematous auditory canal with debris, oedema and exudates
Otitis media	Bulging, erythematous, tympanic membrane (occasionally tympanic membrane yellow)
Tympanic perforation	Direct visualization of the tympanic membrane reveals a tear/hole
Foreign body	Object resting in the external auditory canal

The cardiovascular system

4

Cardinal symptoms	Ischaemic heart disease risk factors	Past investigations/procedures
• Chest pain	• Family history	• ECG
• Dyspnoea	• Smoking	• Exercise tolerance test
• Oedema	• Obesity	• Echocardiogram
• Palpitations	• Diabetes mellitus	• 24-hour ECG tape
• Syncope	• Hypertension	• Angiogram/angioplasty
• Claudication	• Hypercholesterolaemia	• Coronary artery bypass graft

4.1   Canadian Cardiovascular Society

Functional classification of stable angina

Grade 1	Angina with strenuous or rapid or prolonged exertion at work or recreation
Grade 2	Slight limitation of ordinary activity, e.g. walking uphill or walking or climbing stairs rapidly/after meals/in cold/under stress
Grade 3	Marked limitation of ordinary physical activity, e.g. walking 1–2 blocks on the level or climbing < 1 flight of stairs in normal conditions
Grade 4	Inability to carry out any physical activity without discomfort; anginal symptoms at rest

4.2   New York Heart Association

Classification of heart failure symptoms severity

Class 1	No limitations. Ordinary physical activity does not cause undue fatigue, dyspnoea or palpitation
Class 2	Slight limitation of physical activity. Comfortable at rest but ordinary physical activity results in symptoms
Class 3	Marked limitation of physical activity. Less than normal physical activity will lead to symptoms
Class 4	Symptoms of congestive cardiac failure are present at rest. With any physical activity, discomfort is increased

General observations – Breathless at rest, cyanosis

(1) **Hands** – Temperature, peripheral cyanosis, splinter haemorrhages, tar staining, xanthomata

(2) **Radial pulse** – Rate, rhythm, collapsing

(3) **Arm** – Blood pressure, brachial pulse waveform

(4) **Eyes** – Arcus, xanthelasma, anaemia

(5) **Face** – Malar flush

(6) **Lips and tongue** – Central cyanosis

(7) **Neck** – JVP, carotid pulse

(8) **Chest**
Inspection – Scars, pulsations
Palpation – Apex, thrills, heaves
Auscultation – Heart sounds, added sounds, murmurs, carotid bruits, basal crepitations

Other – Radiofemoral synchrony, peripheral pulses, oedema, pulsatile liver, urinalysis

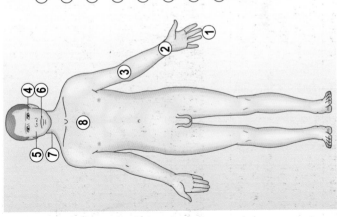

- Inspect the immediate environment: note GTN sprays, heart monitors, infusion pumps and oxygen masks.
- Observe the patient: note breathlessness, distress or anxiety.
- Examine the hands: assess temperature and colour (anaemia, cyanosis), stigmata of endocarditis (splinter haemorrhages and finger clubbing), tar staining (smoker) and tendon xanthomata (raised cholesterol).
- Assess the radial pulses: rate, rhythm and symmetry (see below).
- Look for a collapsing pulse: use the palm of your hand on the elevated, distal forearm. A thumping, pulsing sensation indicates an increased pulse pressure (aortic incompetence/vasodilator therapy) (Fig. 4.1).
- Measure the blood pressure (p. 66).
- Inspect the eyes for corneal arcus and xanthelasma (high cholesterol).
- Look for cyanosis of the tongue, indicative of central cyanosis, and a malar flush, indicative of a low cardiac output.
- Palpate the pulse waveform using the brachial or carotid pulse: press two fingers firmly over the artery; note the character and volume of the pulse (see below).
- Palpate the radial and femoral pulses simultaneously to check for radiofemoral synchrony: in hypertension, absence or delay of the femoral pulse suggests coarctation.

Assessing the pulse

Rate   Normally ranges between 60 and 90/minute; rate > 90 indicates tachycardia and < 60 indicates bradycardia. A *pulse deficit* (pulse rate < heart rate due to non-conducted heart beats) suggests atrial fibrillation.

Rhythm   Normally regular, but quickens during inspiration (sinus arrhythmia). An irregular rhythm is usually due to ectopic beats or atrial fibrillation.

Character of the pulse waveform (larger arteries only)   The normal pulse pressure decreases during inspiration, a change which is clinically apparent and typically exceeds 15 mmHg in severe asthma and pericardial tamponade (*pulsus paradoxus*). A slow-rising, low-volume pulse (*anacrotic pulse*) occurs in aortic stenosis, and a bifid waveform in combined aortic stenosis and incompetence (*pulsus bisferiens*) (Fig. 4.2).

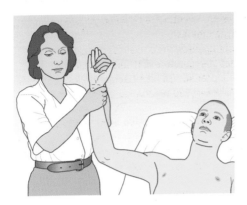

Fig. 4.1 Feeling for a collapsing radial pulse.

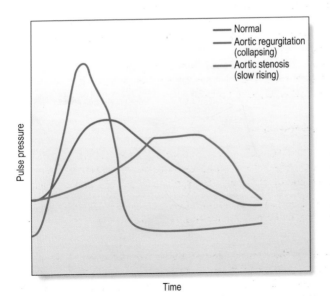

Normal

Aortic regurgitation (collapsing)

Aortic stenosis (slow rising)

Pulse pressure

Time

Fig. 4.2 Character of the three most commonly palpated pulse waveforms.

- Measure the blood pressure with the patient sitting or lying comfortably relaxed, with the upper arm at the level of the heart (Fig. 4.3).
- Choose an inflatable cuff with the appropriate bladder length. For small adults use a 23-cm bladder and for larger adults a 35-cm bladder; too small a bladder length will overestimate the BP and too large a bladder will underestimate the BP.
- Place the centre of the inflatable cuff over the brachial artery and wind the cuff smoothly and firmly around the upper arm.
- If using a mercury sphygmomanometer, check that the mercury reservoir, the cuffed arm and the heart are all at the same level.
- Locate the brachial pulse and inflate the cuff to just over systolic pressure, when the pulse is obliterated.
- Auscultate over the brachial artery while slowly reducing the pressure. Record the systolic pressure when Korotkoff sounds are first heard (phase I) and the diastolic pressure, when sounds disappear (phase V).
- Check the blood pressure after the patient has been standing for several minutes to look for postural hypotension. This is common in patients with salt depletion, autonomic neuropathy, hypotensive drug therapy, or vasovagal syncope.
- If the BP reading is low using an automated sphygmomanometer, check the BP manually.

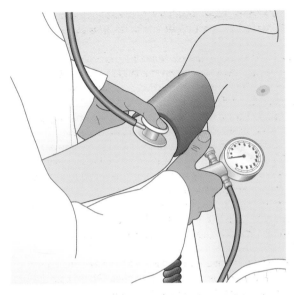

Fig. 4.3   Measuring the blood pressure.

- Position the patient reclining at 45° to the horizontal and ask the patient to turn the head to the left.
- Inspect the root of the neck for pulsations deep to the sternocleidomastoid (Fig. 4.4). Distinguish the carotid artery pulse from internal jugular venous pulsation; the arterial pulse differs from the venous pulse in being outwardly expansile, palpable and does not alter with respiration, patient position or compression of the abdomen.
- Compress the abdomen gently as the patient relaxes the abdominal wall, to identify the internal jugular vein by the visible rise in venous pulsation (*abdominojugular reflux*). If doubt exists, compress the internal jugular vein to distinguish it from an arterial pulsation.
- Measure the vertical height of the JVP above the manubriosternal junction at the peak of the venous pulse (normal < 3 cm) (Fig. 4.5).

JVP waveform (Fig. 4.6)

Persistent elevation of the JVP (3+ cm) is the earliest and most reliable sign of right ventricular failure. The normal JVP has two peaks (a and v) and two troughs (x and y).

The 'a' wave (atrial contraction) is more marked if the pulmonary artery pressure is increased (*giant 'a' waves* suggest pulmonary hypertension). The 'a' waves disappear in the absence of atrial contraction, e.g. atrial fibrillation, and are particularly prominent in atrioventricular dissociation when atrial contraction occurs while the tricuspid valve is closed (*cannon waves*).

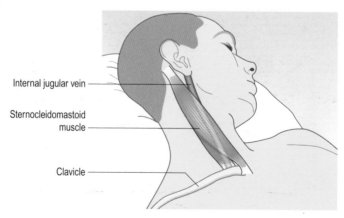

Internal jugular vein

Sternocleidomastoid muscle

Clavicle

   Fig. 4.4 Inspecting the JVP from the side.

The 'v' wave peaks at the end of atrial filling immediately before the tricuspid valve opens. In tricuspid regurgitation, a prominent systolic 'v' wave results from the reflux of blood into the right atrium.

The 'x' trough represents atrial relaxation and the **'y' trough**, the onset of ventricular filling.

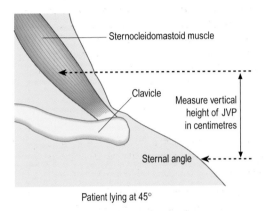

Sternocleidomastoid muscle

Clavicle

Measure vertical height of JVP in centimetres

Sternal angle

Patient lying at 45°

Fig. 4.5 Measuring the height of the JVP.

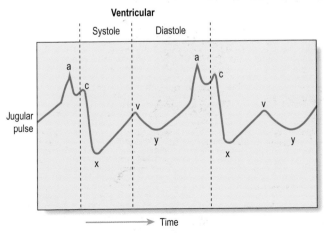

Ventricular

Systole   Diastole

Jugular pulse

Time

Fig. 4.6 Form of the venous pulse wave tracing from the internal jugular vein.

- Inspect the precordium (anterior chest wall): look for scars and implanted pacemakers; look for the apex beat and any other pulsation.
- Palpate the precordium (Fig. 4.7): place the right hand on the left chest wall, localize the apex beat using a finger tip and assess its character as normal, diffuse or heaving (thrusting) (Table 4.3).
- Identify the position of the apex beat (normally in the fifth intercostal space in the midclavicular line; Fig. 4.8) – count the spaces down from the first intercostal space below the clavicle. If the apex beat is difficult to find, roll the patient towards the left side. If the apex beat is displaced, check that the trachea is central (tracheal deviation indicates mediastinal shift).
- Look and feel for a parasternal heave: place the thenar eminence of the right hand on the lower sternum.
- Palpate the anterior chest wall with the patient sitting upright and palpate the apex, in the left lateral position, feel for palpable heart sounds and murmurs (thrills).

The **apex beat** is defined as the furthest point inferiorly and laterally on the chest wall that the finger tip detects a localized cardiac impulse. It is impalpable in 40–50% of individuals and especially in patients with obesity or chronic obstructive pulmonary disease.

4.3 Palpable abnormalities	
Displaced apex	Dilated left ventricle, mediastinal shift
Heaving apex	Left ventricular hypertrophy
Tapping apex	Palpable first heart sound (mitral stenosis)
Double apical impulse	Left ventricular dyskinesia, aneurysm, hypertrophic obstructive cardiomyopathy (HOCM)
Parasternal heave	Right ventricular hypertrophy
Thrill	Palpable murmur (grade 4+)
	Maximal where the murmur is loudest

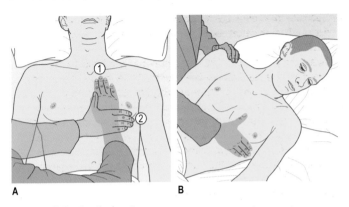

A **B**

Fig. 4.7 Palpating the heart.
(A) Palpate the heart from apex to sternum for parasternal pulsations (1) then use the hand to palpate the apex beat (2). (B) If necessary, roll the patient into the left lateral position.

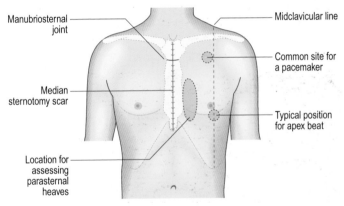

Manubriosternal joint

Midclavicular line

Common site for a pacemaker

Median sternotomy scar

Typical position for apex beat

Location for assessing parasternal heaves

Fig. 4.8 Surface landmarks and signs in the cardiovascular examination.

- Auscultate the four areas using the diaphragm of the stethoscope (aortic, pulmonary, tricuspid and mitral areas shown in Fig. 4.9), then auscultate more widely over the whole precordium and axilla.
- Identify the first and second heart sounds: if necessary, feel the carotid pulse (simultaneous with the first heart sound). The second heart sound is usually softer and higher pitched.
- Listen for added heart sounds and murmurs in the time interval between the heart sounds, with the patient's breath held as necessary.
- Auscultate over both carotid arteries with the patient's breath held, for carotid bruits and aortic systolic murmurs radiating to the carotids.
- Roll the patient on the left side (Fig. 4.10), locate the apex beat and listen both at and lateral to the apex: the pansystolic murmur of mitral incompetence is best heard with the diaphragm; the diastolic murmur of mitral stenosis is best heard with the bell (Fig. 4.2).
- Sit the patient forward and with the patient's breath held in expiration (Fig. 4.10), listen with the diaphragm for the diastolic murmur of aortic incompetence along the left sternal edge.

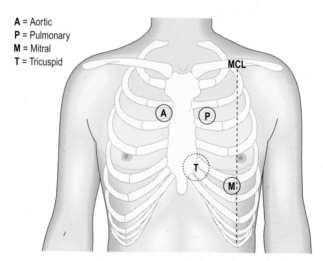

A = Aortic
P = Pulmonary
M = Mitral
T = Tricuspid

Fig. 4.9 Sites for auscultation.
Sites in the neighbourhood of which murmurs from the relevant valves are usually but not always preferentially heard. MCL, midclavicular line.

Using the stethoscope

The diaphragm is designed to amplify high-pitched sounds; the bell does not amplify sound but transmits low-pitched sounds better than the diaphragm. The bell should be placed lightly against the skin; in contrast, the diaphragm should be placed firmly against the skin for optimal sound amplification and transmission. It is possible to make the bell perform like a diaphragm by placing it firmly against the skin, using the skin itself as a diaphragm.

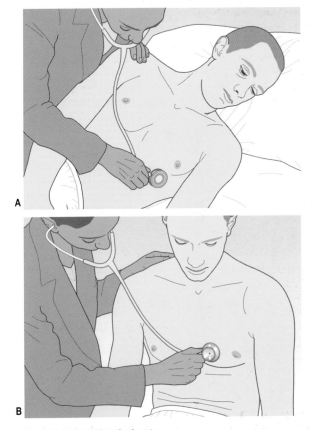

A

B

Fig. 4.10 Auscultating the heart.
(A) Position for mitral stenosis. (B) Position for aortic regurgitation.

The first heart sound (S1) is best heard at the apex and is due to closure of the mitral and tricuspid valves. The intensity is decreased in mitral incompetence and first-degree heart block and increased in mitral stenosis, supraventricular tachycardia, pregnancy and hyperthyroidism.

The second heart sound (S2) is best heard at the left sternal edge in the second or third intercostal space. It is caused by closure of the aortic and pulmonary valves. Delayed closure of the pulmonary valve causes increased splitting of the second heart sound. Splitting during inspiration may be physiological or due to right bundle branch block. Fixed splitting suggests an atrial septal defect. Reversed splitting (occurring in expiration) suggests left bundle branch block.

Added sounds

The third heart sound (S3) imparts a typical cadence to the heart sounds 'lup-dup-dum' – S1–S2–S3. It is commonly heard at the apex in healthy children, young adults and during pregnancy. It occurs during early ventricular filling, is low pitched and best heard using the bell of the stethoscope. It is often present in mitral incompetence and constrictive pericarditis. In the elderly, it signifies cardiac failure.

The fourth heart sound (S4) is coincident with atrial contraction and thus precedes the first heart sound. It is low pitched and imparts a typical cadence to the heart sounds – 'da-lup-dup'. It is often due to hypertension.

An opening snap is pathognomonic of mitral stenosis. It occurs soon after the second heart sound, is high pitched and best heard with the diaphragm between the apex and the left sternal edge.

A pericardial friction rub is characteristic of pericarditis. It is a creaking sound like walking on firm snow, best heard with the patient's breath held. It often has three components sounding like 'chi-te-chi'.

Figure 4.11 shows the relationship of the heart sounds and added sounds to the electrocardiograph and arterial pulse pressure.

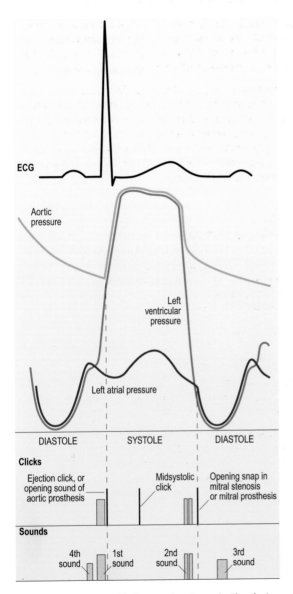

Fig. 4.11 The relationship between heart sounds, the electrocardiogram and the cardiac cycle in the left side of the heart.

Murmurs arise from turbulent blood flow and may occur if a valve is diseased or if there is an increased blood flow through a normal valve. Murmurs can be characterized in the following manner:

- **Site:** the area over which a murmur is best heard depends upon the position of the heart valve or defect and the direction of blood flow (Fig. 4.12).
- **Radiation:** the direction of a murmur's radiation follows the direction of blood flow through the heart valve or cardiac defect.
- **Pitch** may be characteristic. As a rule, the greater the pressure gradient, the higher the pitch. The murmur of mitral stenosis is low pitched and that of aortic incompetence high pitched.
- **Timing:** murmurs are usually either systolic or diastolic (Fig. 4.13); occasionally, murmurs extend through both systole and diastole, e.g. the continuous murmur of a patent ductus arteriosus.
  - *Systole* is defined by the time interval between the first and second heart sounds during which the mitral and tricuspid valves are closed.
  - *Diastole* is defined by the time interval between the second heart sound and the first heart sound during which the aortic and pulmonary valves are closed.
- **Intensity** (Table 4.4): the loudness of a heart murmur is a relatively poor index of its clinical significance.

4.4 Grades of murmur intensity	
Grade 1	Just audible by an expert in optimal conditions
Grade 2	Quiet; just audible by a non-expert in optimal conditions
Grade 3	Moderately loud
Grade 4	Loud and may be accompanied by a palpable thrill
Grade 5	Very loud over a wide area with a palpable thrill
Grade 6	So loud as to be audible without a stethoscope

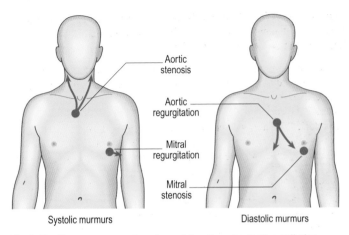

Fig. 4.12 **Murmurs: areas of maximum intensity and selective radiation.**

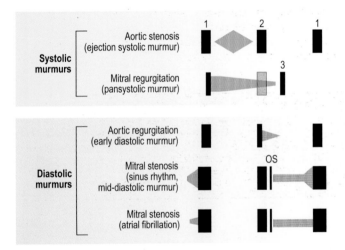

Fig. 4.13 **Representation of timing, pitch and intensity of common murmurs.**
For simplicity, only the mitral component of the first sound and aortic component
of the second sound are illustrated. OS, opening snap.

- Compare the two limbs for evidence of pallor, cyanosis, hair loss and other features of impaired nutrition and blood supply.
- Compare the temperature of the two limbs: use the finger tips and begin in the distal limb and move proximally.
- Check the capillary refilling time after blanching the skin of the toes.
- Locate the dorsalis pedis pulse: place your finger tips immediately lateral to the extensor hallucis longus tendon, proximal to the first metatarsal space (Fig. 4.14A).
- Locate the posterior tibial pulse behind the medial malleolus (Fig. 4.14B).
- Locate the popliteal pulse: place your thumbs on each side of the patellar tendon with the knee slightly flexed and press the finger tips of both hands firmly into the popliteal fossa to palpate the arterial pulse (Fig. 4.14C).
- Palpate the femoral pulse at the mid-inguinal point (Fig. 4.14D); assess the pulse waveform and volume.
- Palpate the radial, brachial and axillary pulses in the upper limbs.
- Check for radiofemoral synchrony, especially in hypertensive patients or patients with suspected aortic dissection.
- Auscultate over the major vessels for bruits (carotid, subclavian, abdominal aorta, renal and femoral arteries) using the diaphragm.
- Feel for an abdominal aortic aneurysm: see page 104.

An arterial bruit indicates turbulent blood flow. It may be audible over, and distal to, the site of stenosis of a major artery, such as the abdominal aorta, the internal carotid, subclavian, femoral or renal arteries. A systolic bruit over the abdominal aorta may be present in a healthy subject. In any patient presenting with hypertension, look for renal bruits suggestive of renovascular hypertension.

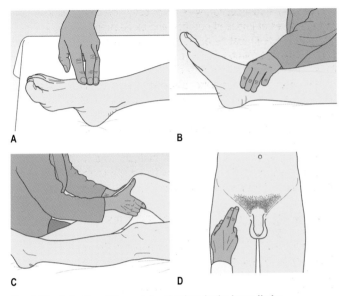

Fig. 4.14 Palpation of the peripheral pulses in the lower limbs.
(A) Dorsalis pedis. (B) Posterior tibial. (C) Popliteal. (D) Femoral.

4.5   Features of chronic lower limb ischaemia

- Pulses – diminished or absent
- Reduced skin temperature
- Loss of hair
- Muscle atrophy
- Guttering of superficial veins (veins empty on minimal elevation of the leg)
- Pallor on elevation with delayed reddening on dependency

4.6   The 6 Ps of acute limb ischaemia

- Pain
- Pallor
- Pulselessness
- Perishing cold
- Paraesthesia
- Paralysis

Deep vein thrombosis

- Compare the colour of both legs and look for evidence of blanching or cyanosis of the skin and toenails.
- Look for venous distension: check if the superficial veins empty promptly on elevation of the limb.
- Gently palpate the calf for evidence of heat and tenderness but avoid unnecessary compression of the calf muscles.
- Feel for tenderness overlying the femoral vein.
- Look for pitting oedema at the ankle; note its extent up the leg.
- Measure the calf diameter of the leg: use a tape measure to compare the two legs at a fixed distance from the medial malleolus.

Saphenofemoral venous incompetence (Trendelenburg's test)

- Elevate the leg with the patient lying supine.
- Compress the superficial veins using a tourniquet in the upper thigh.
- Look for venous filling as the patient stands upright.
- Release the tourniquet and watch the veins fill.

If the superficial veins fill slowly on standing but rapidly on releasing the tourniquet, an incompetent saphenofemoral valve is likely. However, filling of the veins regardless of tourniquet pressure is due to incompetence of one or more of the valves of the deep perforating veins. Identify the level of valve incompetence by repositioning the tourniquet at the levels shown in Figure 4.15 and repeating the above sequence.

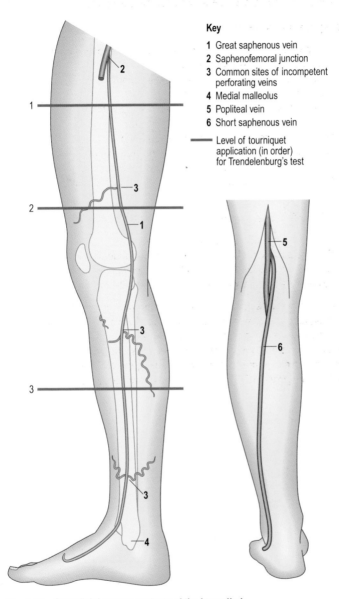

Key

1 Great saphenous vein
2 Saphenofemoral junction
3 Common sites of incompetent perforating veins
4 Medial malleolus
5 Popliteal vein
6 Short saphenous vein

— Level of tourniquet application (in order) for Trendelenburg's test

Fig. 4.15 Superficial venous anatomy of the lower limb

The respiratory system

Cardinal symptoms	Risk factors for factor	Asthma trigger DVT/PE
• Dyspnoea*	• Past history DVT/PE	• Allergens (house dust mite, pets, pollen, moulds)
• Cough	• Family history DVT/PE	• Cigarette smoke
• Sputum	• Surgery (especially pelvic/orthopaedic)	• Cold air
• Haemoptysis	• Immobility	• Infection (e.g. viral URTI)
• Wheeze	• Pregnancy/oral contraceptive	• Exercise
• Pleuritic pain	• Malignancy	• Drugs (NSAIDs, beta-blockers)
	• Thrombophilia	• Poor drug compliance
	• Obesity	

*Ask about smoking, home oxygen therapy, home nebuliser therapy and the patient's normal peak flow rate.

5.1 Respiratory causes of breathlessness

Sudden (seconds/minutes)	Pulmonary embolism, Pneumothorax, acute asthma
Acute (hours/days)	Pneumonia, Exacerbation of COPD
Intermediate (days/weeks)	Pleural effusion, Bronchial carcinoma, Pulmonary tuberculosis
Chronic (months/years)	COPD, bronchiectasis, Fibrosing alveolitis

5.2 Sputum

Type	Appearance	Cause
Serous	Clear, watery, frothy (may be pink)	Pulmonary oedema
Mucoid	Clear, grey, white, may be black (soot)	COPD, chronic asthma
Purulent	Yellow, green brown	Bacterial infection
Rusty	Rusty, golden yellow	Pneumococcal pneumonia

General observations – Inhalers, oxygen therapy, anaemia, sputum, breathlessness, stridor, cachexia

① **Hands** – Clubbing, flapping tremor, tar stain, cyanosis, bounding pulse, small muscle wasting

② **Head and neck** – Horner's/Pancoast's syndrome, SVC obstruction, chemosis, cyanosis, JVP, lymphadenopathy, tracheal position, SLE rash

③ **Chest (posterior then anterior)**
Inspection – Scars, lesions, chest shape, respiratory rate, chest expansion, peak flow
Palpation – Chest expansion
Percussion – Entire chest
Auscultation – Breath sounds, vocal resonance

④ **Genitalia** – Testicular tumour

⑤ **Legs** – Pitting oedema, DVT, toe clubbing, erythema nodosum

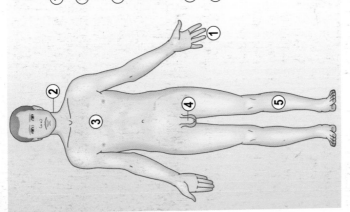

- Inspect the patient's immediate environment: note inhalers, content of sputum pots, oxygen mask, nebulizers and pulse oximeter.
- Observe the patient: note evidence of cachexia, breathlessness, wheeze or stridor. Look for the features of superior vena caval (SVC) obstruction and Pancoast's syndrome if bronchial carcinoma is suspected.
- Measure the respiratory rate: feel the radial pulse to distract the patient's attention whilst counting the respiratory rate.
- Examine the hands: look for tar staining and finger clubbing.
- Look for a flapping tremor (*asterixis*): ask the patient to extend both arms and cock the wrists back.
- Look for evidence of cyanosis: central and/or peripheral cyanosis (p. 64).
- Examine the jugular venous pressure (JVP): note its height above the manubriosternal junction and whether or not it is pulsatile (p. 68).
- Palpate for lymphadenopathy (Fig. 5.1) beneath the mandible, in the anterior and posterior triangles of the neck and above the clavicles.

Stridor is a high-pitched, crowing sound that occurs during inspiration and is accentuated by coughing. It is a feature of upper airways obstruction (either laryngeal or tracheal) requiring urgent assessment.

Superior vena caval (SVC) obstruction is suggested by non-pulsatile, distended jugular veins, dilated, superficial venules on the face and chest wall, facial oedema and chemosis (conjunctival oedema).

Pancoast's syndrome is due to apical lung tumour resulting in pain in the arm and hand, small muscle wasting of the hand, sympathetic palsy with pupil constriction (Horner's) and SVC obstruction.

Asterixis (Fig. 5.2) is a repetitive, jerky tremor of the outstretched hands resulting in transient loss of extensor muscle tone at the wrist. It is due to a metabolic brain stem dysfunction and is common in ventilatory failure, hepatic encephalopathy, renal failure and cardiac failure.

Central cyanosis (blue tongue, lips and fingers with warm hands) results from a *central* failure of oxygen transfer across the lung alveolar–capillary membranes; also seen in polycythaemia due to excess deoxygenated haemoglobin or to abnormal haemoglobins, e.g. methaemoglobin and sulphaemoglobin. **Peripheral cyanosis** (cold, blue fingers) results from *peripheral* circulatory failure causing excessive oxygen extraction from the capillaries.

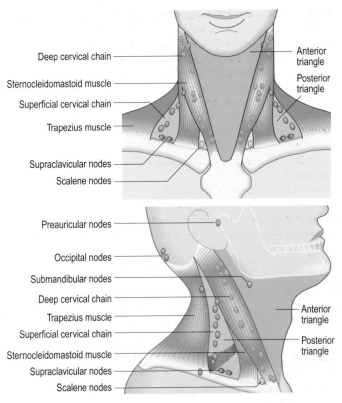

Deep cervical chain

Sternocleidomastoid muscle

Superficial cervical chain

Trapezius muscle

Supraclavicular nodes

Scalene nodes

Anterior triangle

Posterior triangle

Preauricular nodes

Occipital nodes

Submandibular nodes

Deep cervical chain

Trapezius muscle

Superficial cervical chain

Sternocleidomastoid muscle

Supraclavicular nodes

Scalene nodes

Anterior triangle

Posterior triangle

Fig. 5.1 Anatomy of deep and superficial cervical lymphatic chains.

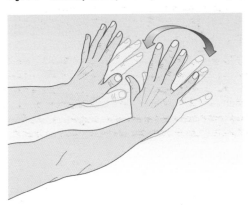

Fig. 5.2 Hand and arm position for observing asterixis.

- Observe the chest: ask the patient to put the arms behind the neck to examine the front and sides of the chest and axillae, and to cross the arms to examine the back of the chest.
- Look for: scars, venous dilatation on the chest wall, metastatic skin deposits and abnormalities of the chest shape (Figs 5.3 and 5.4).
- Observe the respiratory movements: note the depth, pattern and symmetry of respiratory movements both at rest and during deep inspiration.
- Assess the mode of respiration: look for pursed-lip breathing, abdominal rather than chest wall movement and intercostal muscle indrawing (*Hoover's sign*), all features of chronic obstructive pulmonary disease (COPD).
- Measure peak expiratory flow rate by asking the patient to breath as forcefully as possible through a peak flow meter after deep inspiration. Record the best of three attempts.
- Measure the chest expansion: use a tape measure at the level of the fourth intercostal space and record the difference in chest circumference between inspiration and expiration (normally 5+ cm) (Table 5.3).

Features of respiration

Depth Only marked degrees of hyper- or hypoventilation are detectable. The former may be apparent in metabolic acidosis or anxiety ('air hunger') and the latter in opiate toxicity.

Pattern The presence of alternating apnoea and hyperpnoea is known as 'Cheyne–Stokes' breathing – seen in brain stem ischaemia and severe left ventricular failure (altered CO_2 sensitivity of respiratory centre).

Mode Normally, breathing is 75% diaphragmatic (abdominal) and 25% thoracic; thoracic expansion can be limited by pleuritic pain and diaphragmatic contraction by peritonitis or abdominal distension. Pursed-lip breathing, often present in COPD, is ergonomically a more effective means of expiration.

Peak expiratory flow rate (PEFR) provides a useful estimate of airway calibre in obstructive airways disease, e.g. asthma and COPD.

5.3 Features of hyperinflation
- Increased AP diameter
- Decreased cricosternal distance
- Decreased chest expansion < 5 cm
- Intercostal muscle indrawing (Hoover's sign)

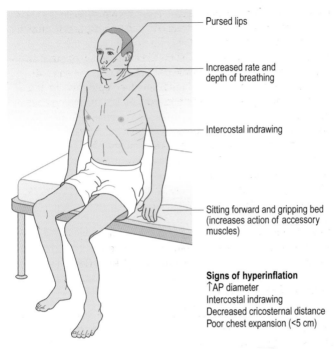

Pursed lips

Increased rate and depth of breathing

Intercostal indrawing

Sitting forward and gripping bed (increases action of accessory muscles)

Signs of hyperinflation
↑AP diameter
Intercostal indrawing
Decreased cricosternal distance
Poor chest expansion (<5 cm)

Fig. 5.3 Features of COPD.

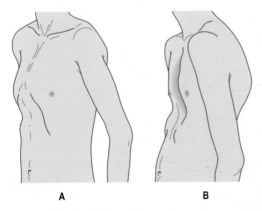

A   B

Fig. 5.4 Chest wall deformities.
(A) Pectus excavatum. (B) Pectus carinatum.

- Check the centrality of the trachea: insert the tip of the index finger into the suprasternal notch, allowing it to slip to either side of the trachea (Fig. 5.5A). Does the finger tip fit more easily into one or other side of the trachea? Check the position of the apex beat to confirm or exclude mediastinal displacement.
- Measure the cricosternal distance: locate the cricoid cartilage below the larynx and insert the finger tips vertically between the cricoid and the suprasternal notch after full inspiration (normal c. 5 cm) (Fig. 5.5B).
- Palpate for symmetry of respiratory movements: place both hands firmly on the chest wall. Assess the movement between the hands as the patient breathes in deeply; perform on both the anterior and the posterior chest wall (Fig. 5.6).

The trachea may be displaced towards the side of a pneumothorax, lung collapse or upper lobe fibrosis or displaced away from a tension pneumothorax or large pleural effusion.

A cricosternal distance of less than the equivalent of three of the patient's finger breadths indicates hyperinflation; this is often apparent as a visible 'descent' of the trachea during inspiration (*tracheal tug*).

Unilaterally reduced chest expansion indicates pathology on that side. Symmetrical reduction in chest expansion is commonly seen in asthma and COPD. The symmetry and degree of chest expansion are more reliably assessed by observation of respiratory movements than by palpation of the chest wall.

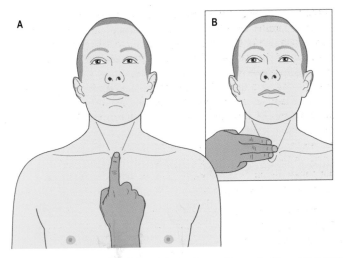

Fig. 5.5 Identifying the position of the trachea and assessing the cricosternal distance.

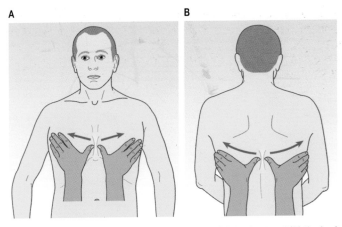

Fig. 5.6 Assessing respiratory movements from (A) the front and (B) the back.

- Percuss the chest: place one hand on the chest wall with the fingers slightly separated. Press the middle finger firmly into the intercostal space to be percussed.
- Strike the centre of the middle phalanx of the middle finger sharply with the tip of the middle finger. The middle finger should be held in partial flexion and the entire movement should come from the wrist.
- Compare the note at equivalent sites on the two sides (Fig. 5.7). When an area of altered resonance is found, map out its boundaries by percussing from areas of normal resonance to areas of dullness.

Common percussion notes (Table 5.4)

Percussion notes across the chest vary with the density of the underlying structures. Percussion may be helpful in determining the position of organs and the presence of masses or fluid (Fig. 5.8).

5.4 Causes of different percussion notes	
Note	**Cause**
Dull	Liver, spleen, heart, lung consolidation/collapse
Resonant	Air-filled lung
Stony dull	Pleural effusion/thickening
Hyperresonant	Emphysema, pneumothorax
Tympanitic	Gas-filled viscus

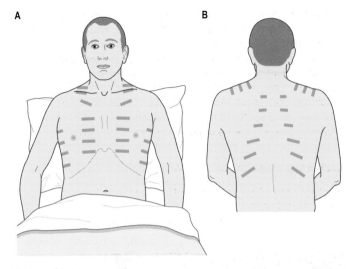

Fig. 5.7 Sites for percussion.
(A) Anterior and lateral chest wall. (B) Posterior chest wall.

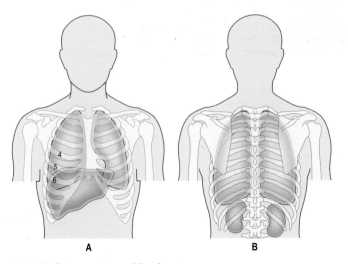

Fig. 5.8 Surface anatomy of the viscera.
(A) Anterior. (B) Posterior.

- Listen to the breath sounds: ask the patient to breathe in and out through an open mouth; use the diaphragm (or the bell if the patient is thin and has prominent ribs preventing good skin contact).
- Compare the breath sounds: listen over equivalent positions on each side of the chest and compare the volume and character of the sounds.
- Characterize the breath sounds: note the volume, quality (timbre) and duration of breath sounds and compare inspiration with expiration.
- Assess vocal resonance: ask the patient to say 'ninety-nine' and compare the sounds transmitted at equivalent positions on each side.

Breath sounds are produced by vibrations of the vocal cords caused by air flow during inspiration and expiration. The sounds are transmitted along the trachea and bronchi, through the lung parenchyma to the chest wall. Sound travels best through solid media rather than air; in consequence, pathological processes of the lung and surrounding tissues change the volume and frequency of transmitted sound, generating characteristic clinical signs. Breath sounds are normally *vesicular* (Fig. 5.9A) but may become diminished vesicular or *bronchial* (Fig. 5.9B). Bronchial breath sounds are louder and harsher breath sounds occurring in *both* inspiration and expiration; when present, they indicate lung consolidation in the presence of patent airways.

Vocal resonance, like the breath sounds, reflects changes in lung density and airway patency and can help identify underlying disease. Resonance is increased in consolidation of the lung and decreased in lung collapse (due to airway occlusion).

Additional sounds occur in the presence of significant lung disorders such as *rhonchi* in small airways obstruction, *crackles (crepitations)* in interstitial lung disease or a *pleural rub* in pleuropericardial inflammatory disorders (Table 5.5).

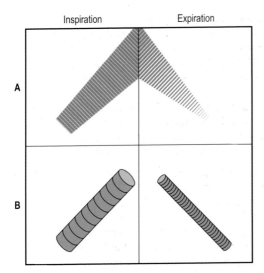

Fig. 5.9A Vesicular breath sounds.
The intensity of these sounds increases steadily during inspiration, then quickly fades away during the first third of expiration.

Fig. 5.9B Bronchial breath sounds.
There are three criteria for bronchial breath sounds: (1) Inspiratory and expiratory sounds are loud and blowing; (2) The expiratory sound is as long and as loud as the inspiratory sound; (3) There is an audible pause between inspiration and expiration.

5.5 Added sounds	
Rhonchi (wheezes)	High-pitched musical sounds produced by air passing through narrowed airways, e.g. asthma
Crackles (crepitations)	Non-musical sounds during inspiration caused by the reopening of occluded airways, e.g. pulmonary oedema
Pleural friction rub	Leathery or creaking sounds produced by movement of roughened pleural surfaces over each other, e.g. pleurisy caused by pneumonia

5.6 The interpretation of signs in respiratory disease

Abnormality	Chest wall movement	Mediastinal displacement	Percussion note	Breath sounds	Vocal resonance	Added sounds
Consolidation	Decreased on affected side	None	Dull	Bronchial	Increased	Crepitations
Collapse	Decreased on affected side	Towards affected side	Dull	Decreased or absent	Decreased or absent	None
Effusion	Decreased on affected side	Towards opposite side	Stony dull	Decreased or absent	Decreased or absent	May be pleural rub
Pneumothorax	Decreased on affected side	Towards opposite side	Normal or hyperresonant	Decreased or absent	Decreased or absent	None
Emphysema	Decreased on both sides	None	Normal or hyperresonant	Decreased	Normal or decreased	None
Asthma	Decreased on both sides	None	Normal or hyperresonant	Prolonged expiration	Normal	Rhonchi

The gastrointestinal and genitourinary systems

Cardinal symptoms (GI)	Cardinal symptoms (GU)	Previous investigations
• Dysphagia	• Dysuria/urgency	• Upper GI endoscopy
• Nausea and vomiting	• Haematuria	• Colonoscopy
• Heartburn	• Frequency/nocturia	• Barium studies
• Abdominal pain	• Hesitancy/poor stream	• Abdominal/renal ultrasound
• Anorexia/weight loss	• Urinary incontinence	• Liver/renal biopsy
• Altered bowel habit	• Urethral/vaginal discharge	• Intravenous urogram
• Rectal bleeding	• Menstrual problems	• Cystoscopy
• Jaundice	• Sexual problems	• Cervical screening

6.1 Systemic features of inflammatory bowel disease

General	Fever, malaise, weight loss
Eyes	Conjunctivitis, episcleritis, iritis
Joints	Arthralgia of large joints, Sacroiliitis/ankylosing spondylitis
Skin	Mouth ulcers, erythema nodosum, Pyoderma gangrenosum
Liver	Fatty liver, gallstones, Sclerosing cholangitis
Cholangiocarcinoma (UC) Renal	Oxalate stones, amyloidosis (rare)

6.2 Common presenting features of alcoholism

- Accidents and trauma
- Obesity and diabetes mellitus
- Dyspepsia
- Diarrhoea
- Hepatitis and pancreatitis
- Infertility and fetal damage
- Osteoporosis, psoriasis
- Blackouts and seizures
- Hypertension and arrhythmias
- Stroke, brain damage and neuropathy

General observations – BMI, waist circumference, nutrition, jaundice

(1) **Hands** – Clubbing, palmar erythema, Dupuytren's contracture, liver flap, nail changes

(2) **Eyes** – Sclera (colour), conjunctiva (pallor)

(3) **Head and neck** – Spider naevi, dentition, fetor hepaticus, JVP

(4) **Chest** – Gynaecomastia, spider naevi

(5) **Abdomen**
Inspection – Scars, distension, masses, peristalsis, movement (with respiration), venous distension
Palpation – Superficial, deep, liver, spleen, kidneys, bladder, aorta
Percussion – Liver, spleen, bladder, shifting dullness
Auscultation – Bowel sounds, bruits

(6) **Hernial orifices** – Lymph nodes, genitalia

Other – Urinalysis, faecal occult blood, leg oedema

- Observe the patient: look for evidence of malnutrition, dehydration (skin turgor) and jaundice, and smell the breath for fetor hepaticus – a characteristic sickly sweet smell in hepatic failure.
- Examine the nails and hands: look for leukonychia (white nails), koilonychia (spoon-shaped nails), finger clubbing, palmar erythema (mottled redness over the hypothenar eminence) and Dupuytren's contracture (thickening and contracture of the palmar fascia) (Table 6.3).
- Check for asterixis: ask the patient to extend both arms, cock the wrists back and look for a flapping tremor (see p. 87).
- Inspect the upper limbs for tattoos, stigmata of IV drug abuse, scratch marks (pruritus), spider naevi and loss of axillary hair.
- Gently retract the lower eyelid: check for conjunctival pallor (anaemia) and look at the sclera for jaundice.
- Examine the mouth, tongue and teeth: use a torch and tongue depressor to look at the teeth and buccal mucosa for ulcers or thrush. The tongue appears smooth and clean-looking in atrophic glossitis due to iron, folate or vitamin B_{12} deficiency.
- Examine the face, neck and upper chest for spider naevi (Table 6.4).
- Palpate for supraclavicular lymph nodes.
- Examine the male breasts: gynaecomastia occurs in liver disease.
- Look at the lower limbs: note any skin rashes (dermatitis herpetiformis in coeliac disease, pyoderma in inflammatory bowel disease) and look for ankle oedema.

Malignant lymphadenopathy arising from upper gastrointestinal tumours usually occurs in the left supraclavicular fossa (Troisier's sign – Virchow's node) due to spread along the thoracic duct.

6.3 Signs of chronic liver disease

Finger clubbing	Gynaecomastia
Leukonychia	Testicular atrophy
Palmar erythema	Loss of axillary hair
Dupuytren's contracture	Parotid enlargement
Spider naevi	Peripheral oedema

6.4 Spider naevi (central arteriole with branches)

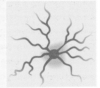

- Five or more suggests liver disease
- Occur in the territory of the superior vena cava, i.e. hands, face, neck, upper chest and back
- Blanch when pressure is applied to the central arteriole, refilling from the centre outwards.
- Differ from Campbell de Morgan spots (of no clinical significance) which do *not* blanch on pressure

6.5 West Haven grading of hepatic encephalopathy

Stage	Alteration of consciousness
Stage 0	No change in personality or behaviour – no asterixis
Stage 1	Impaired concentration and attention span Sleep disturbance, slurred speech, asterixis, agitation or depression
Stage 2	Lethargy, drowsiness, apathy or aggression Disorientation. Inappropriate behaviour. Slurred speech
Stage 3	Confusion and disorientation. Bizarre behaviour Drowsiness or stupor. Asterixis is usually absent
Stage 4	Comatose with no response to voice commands Minimal or absent response to painful stimuli

6.6 Child – Pugh classification of prognosis in cirrhosis

Score	1	2	3
Bilirubin (µmol/L)	< 34	34–50	> 50
Albumin (g/L)	> 35	28–35	< 28
Ascites	None	Mild	Marked
Encephalopathy	None	Mild	Marked
Prothrombin Time (seconds)	< 4	4–6	> 6

Child A = Score < 7   1 year survival 82%
Child B = Score 7–9   1 year survival 62%
Child C = Score > 9   1 year survival 42%

- Position the patient supine with the head resting on one pillow and arms by the sides in order to relax the abdominal musculature.
- Expose the abdomen from xiphisternum to symphysis pubis.
- Inspect the abdomen: note its shape and symmetry, surgical scars and stomas.
- Observe: any movement with respiration, visible pulsations, peristalsis, masses, striae and distended veins.
- Ask about any pain or discomfort before palpating the abdomen, then begin palpation at a site remote from the area of pain.
- Lightly palpate the areas shown in Figure 6.1 using gentle dipping motions of the hand, without breaking contact with the skin.
- Assess muscle tone in each area and look at the patient's expressions, checking for any signs of discomfort. If appropriate, look for rebound tenderness by abruptly removing the palpating hand.
- Palpate more deeply, pressing firmly in each region and characterize any mass found (Fig. 6.2) using the system detailed on page 52.

Guarding   Reflex contraction of the abdominal muscles on light palpation, often associated with localized pain, due to inflammation of the parietal peritoneum.

Rebound tenderness   Pain caused by the sudden withdrawal of a firmly applied hand on the abdominal wall; though a non-specific feature, it suggests the presence of an underlying inflamed viscus.

Rigidity   Spasm of the abdominal muscles associated with peritonitis; if severe, the abdomen may be board-like. It often disappears despite subsequent progression of the inflammatory process.

Visible peristalsis   Gastric peristalsis may be seen in gastric outlet obstruction (pyloric stenosis); it appears as a slow wave of contraction passing from left to right from the left hypochondrium across the midline. A dilated, obstructed stomach forms a prominent swelling in the upper abdomen; gentle shaking of the patient to elicit a 'succussion splash' two or more hours after a meal, suggests pyloric obstruction.

A sunken, **scaphoid abdomen** may be due to profound weight loss.

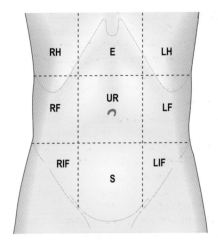

RH	**E**	**LH**
RF	**UR**	**LF**
RIF	**S**	**LIF**

RH Right hypochondrium
LH Left hypochondrium
 E Epigastrium
RF Right flank
LF Left flank
UR Umbilical region
RIF Right iliac fossa
LIF Left iliac fossa
 S Suprapubic region
or hypogastrium

Fig. 6.1   Regions of the abdomen.

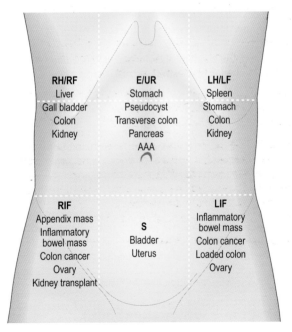

RH/RF	**E/UR**	**LH/LF**
Liver	Stomach	Spleen
Gall bladder	Pseudocyst	Stomach
Colon	Transverse colon	Colon
Kidney	Pancreas	Kidney
	AAA	

RIF	**S**	**LIF**
Appendix mass		Inflammatory
Inflammatory	Bladder	bowel mass
bowel mass	Uterus	Colon cancer
Colon cancer		Loaded colon
Ovary		Ovary
Kidney transplant		

Fig. 6.2   Sites of abdominal masses and their possible cause.

- Palpate the *liver* (Fig. 6.3): place a hand flat on the abdominal wall in the right midclavicular line, so that the finger tips lie perpendicular to the costal margin. As the patient breathes in deeply, gently depress the hand into the abdomen until the finger tips detect the liver edge at the height of inspiration. Start in the flank, moving towards the costal margin with each inspiration, until the liver is felt or the costal margin is reached.
- Trace the surface and edge of a palpable liver across the abdomen; note its shape, size (in cm below costal margin), texture and any tenderness or pulsatility.
- Look for tenderness overlying an inflamed *gall bladder*: press the thumb under the costal margin in the midclavicular line and ask the patient to breathe in deeply; note any sudden arrest of inspiration because of localized pain (*Murphy's sign*)
- Palpate the *spleen* (Fig. 6.4): place a hand flat on the abdominal wall perpendicular to the left costal margin with the finger tips at the umbilicus. As the patient breathes in deeply, gently depress the hand into the abdomen until the finger tips detect the splenic edge at the height of inspiration. Move the hand towards the costal margin with each inspiration, until the spleen is felt or the costal margin is reached.
- Palpate the *kidneys*: use a bimanual technique with one hand behind the flank and the other just beneath the costal margin in the midclavicular line (Fig. 6.5). Ask the patient to breathe in deeply as the two hands gently close on the kidney. At maximal inspiration, try to flip the kidney up from below, between the two hands (ballotting).
- Palpate the *aorta*: place the forefinger and thumb of one hand on either side of the midline in the epigastrium. Press down firmly until a pulsation is felt; assessing the diameter of the aorta by palpation is unreliable and if doubt exists, an ultrasound scan should be done.

The normal spleen lies deep to ribs 9–11 and never extends beyond the midaxillary line. Splenic enlargement causes dullness to percussion over the spleen, extending into the lower chest; it is best distinguished from an enlarged kidney by percussion, movement on respiration and the inability to palpate between it and the costal margin (Table 6.7).

6.7   Features distinguishing the spleen from the kidney on palpation
• The spleen moves early on respiration • Dullness to percussion over the spleen (resonance over the kidney) • Inability to palpate between the spleen and the costal margin

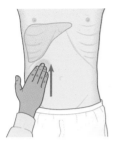

Fig. 6.3   Palpation of the liver.

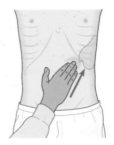

Fig. 6.4   Palpation of the spleen.

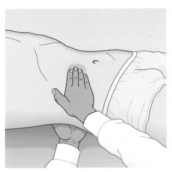

Right   Left

Fig. 6.5   Palpation of the kidneys.

6.8 Causes of hepatic and splenic enlargement		
Hepatomegaly	**Splenomegaly**	**Hepatosplenomegaly**
Congestive heart failure	Portal hypertension	Myelofibrosis
Alcoholic hepatitis	Haemolytic anaemia	Lymphoma
Viral hepatitis	Infection (e.g. malaria, endocarditis)	Cirrhosis
Hepatocellular cancer	SLE and RA	Sarcoidosis
Hepatic metastases		Amyloidosis

- Percuss from areas of resonance to dullness to define the extent of any mass or organomegaly found.
- Percuss the upper and lower borders of the liver and spleen and around the bladder, pelvic organs and any masses found.
- Look for *shifting dullness* if there is any abdominal distension (Fig. 6.6).
- Percuss from the midline to the flanks and symphysis pubis until the percussion note changes from tympanitic to dull.
- Mark the boundary between the area of resonance and dullness; roll the patient towards you and wait 10 seconds for the fluid to redistribute.
- Percuss again: if the percussion note in the flank changes from resonant to dull, confirm the finding by percussing back towards the midline, which should still be resonant.
- Listen for bowels sounds for at least 1 minute (Table 6.9).
- Listen over the aorta and renal arteries for bruits.
- Try to elicit a *succussion splash* if gastric outlet obstruction is suspected; place one hand under the ribcage in each flank and shake the patient vigorously from side to side.

Ascites (Table 6.10) is suggested by central resonance with dullness in the flanks and pelvis (*shifting dullness*); in contrast, pelvic masses cause displacement of bowel to the flanks, resulting in central dullness and flank resonance.

Abdominal distension may be apparent to the patient yet undetectable by the observer (*functional bloating*). Visible distension may be caused by *fat*, *flatus*, *faeces*, *fetus*, *fluid* and *functional bloating*. Exclude the possibilities of increased abdominal wall fat by assessing the thickness of the subcutaneous tissues on gently pinching, or by observing the shape of the abdomen as the patient sits forward.

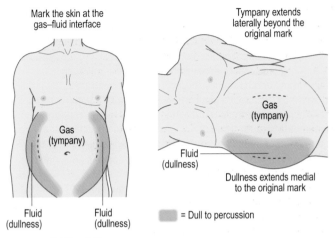

Mark the skin at the gas–fluid interface

Gas (tympany)

Fluid (dullness)   Fluid (dullness)

Tympany extends laterally beyond the original mark

Gas (tympany)

Fluid (dullness)

Dullness extends medial to the original mark

= Dull to percussion

Fig. 6.6 Shifting dullness.

6.9 Bowel sounds	
Gurgling every 10–20 s	Normal
Increased activity	Normal/gastroenteritis
High pitched + tinkling	Mechanical obstruction
Absence of sounds	Paralytic ileus

6.10 Causes of ascites	
Exudates (protein > 30 g/L)	**Transudates (protein < 30 g/L)**
Carcinomatosis	Cirrhosis with portal hypertension
Pancreatitis	Congestive heart failure
Infection (including TB)	Nephrotic syndrome
Inferior vena cava (IVC)/hepatic vein obstruction	Portal vein thrombosis
Hypothyroidism	

- Inspect the inguinal regions and scrotum: ask the patient to stand, expose the groin fully and look for an inguinal swelling.
- Ask the patient to cough: look for movement in the inguinal region and feel for a cough impulse over the inguinal canals and scrotum.
- Note the characteristics of any hernia: check the size, colour, temperature and tenderness of any swelling; identify its relationship to the pubic tubercle to identify the type of hernia (Table 6.11).
- Ask the patient to try to reduce the hernia by gently 'massaging' the hernia back into the abdomen.
- If reducible, occlude the deep inguinal ring: apply pressure at the mid-inguinal point and check if the hernia reappears on coughing.
- Examine the penis and palpate the testes, epididymes and spermatic cords: assess any swelling as previously described (p. 52).
- Check the origin of any swelling: ensure that the mass is not a scrotal swelling (p. 112).

A mass with an expansile cough impulse is a hernia. Femoral hernias lie below and lateral to the pubic tubercle; inguinal hernias lie above and medial to the pubic tubercle (Fig. 6.7).

An irreducible hernia may become *obstructed* when the bowel lumen is occluded and subsequently, *strangulated* if its vascular supply is impaired. A **strangulated hernia** is hot, tense and tender, shows no impulse on coughing and requires immediate surgical attention.

A hydrocele is cystic in nature and usually transilluminates; it is best differentiated from a spermatocele or an epididymal cyst by its relationship to the testis. If in doubt, an ultrasound scan is indicated.

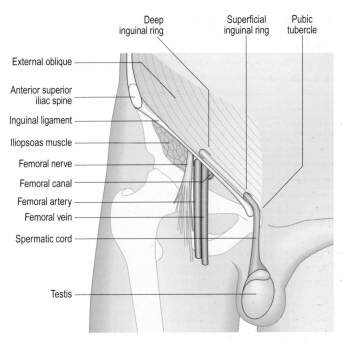

Fig. 6.7 Anatomy of the inguinal canal.

6.11 Hernias		
Indirect inguinal	**Direct inguinal**	**Femoral**
Commonly into scrotum	Rarely into scrotum	Never into scrotum
Has cough impulse	Has cough impulse	Rarely has cough impulse
Can be very large	Moderate size	Normally 3–5 cm diameter
Superior to pubic tubercle	Superior to pubic tubercle	Inferior to pubic tubercle
Can be reduced	Almost always reducible	Rarely reducible
Controlled by deep inguinal ring pressure	Not controlled by deep inguinal ring pressure	Not controlled by deep inguinal ring pressure

- Obtain the patient's informed consent: offer a chaperone.
- Reassure the patient: rectal examination may be uncomfortable but it should not be painful.
- Place the patient in the left lateral position: ask the patient to place the buttocks at the edge of the couch with the knees drawn up.
- Use lidocaine (lignocaine) gel in the anal canal if an anal fissure is suspected.
- Use gloves: examine the perianal skin in a good light, looking for evidence of skin lesions, external haemorrhoids or fistulas.
- Lubricate the examining forefinger.
- Place the tip of the forefinger on the anal margin and with steady pressure on the sphincter, pass the finger gently through the anal canal into the rectum (Fig. 6.8A and B).
- Ask the patient to squeeze the examining forefinger with the anal sphincter; note the strength and symmetry of sphincter contraction.
- Palpate around the entire circumference of the rectum; note any abnormality and assess any mass systematically.
- Repeat the rectal examination after the patient has defecated, if in doubt about palpable masses.
- Examine the finger after withdrawal for the presence of blood and mucus; test the stool sample for blood using a 'Haemoccult' kit.

The rectum is normally empty, with smooth, soft walls. The coccyx and sacrum can be felt through the posterior rectal wall. In the female, the cervix uteri can be felt as a firm, round mass anteriorly (Fig. 6.8C). Vaginal tampons or a pessary may also be felt, confusing the novice. In the male, the prostate is felt anteriorly (Fig. 6.8D).

The normal prostate gland is smooth with a firm consistency, its contours are like miniature buttocks represented by a shallow median groove between the lateral lobes. Pain and tenderness over the prostate suggests prostatitis. Symmetrical enlargement suggests benign hypertrophy; asymmetrical enlargement suggests carcinoma of the prostate.

Clinical errors result from failure to perform rectal examinations. *'If you don't put your finger in it, you may put your foot in it!'*

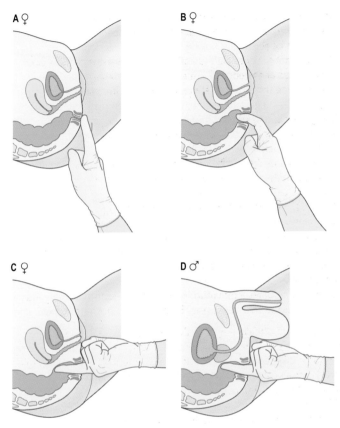

Fig. 6.8 Rectal examination.

- Obtain the patient's informed consent and offer a chaperone.
- Position the patient supine with legs apart: inspect the genitalia, groins and upper thighs looking for rashes or infestation.
- Ask the patient to retract his foreskin to examine the prepuce and glans penis for evidence of rashes, ulcers and discharges.
- Wear gloves and use both hands to palpate each testis in turn between forefinger and thumb; identify the spermatic cord and epididymis and assess any irregularity, swelling or tenderness.
- Confirm that any scrotal swelling originates in the scrotum and is not an inguinal hernia.
- Transilluminate any scrotal swelling using a pen-torch to identify whether the swelling is solid or cystic.

Examination of the genitalia is important but is often omitted to avoid mutual embarrassment. In young males presenting with acute abdominal pain, torsion of the testis can cause abdominal pain, and delayed diagnosis may result in testicular infarction and loss of the testicle. Pain, swelling and redness of the testicle may result from epididymitis, orchitis or torsion of the testicle.

Hydroceles usually transilluminate, unlike spermatoceles (small epididymal cysts) and varicoceles (varicose veins in the spermatic cord, which feel like 'a bag of worms') (Fig. 6.9). A hydrocele may obscure a testicular tumour; if in doubt, an ultrasound scan of the testis is indicated.

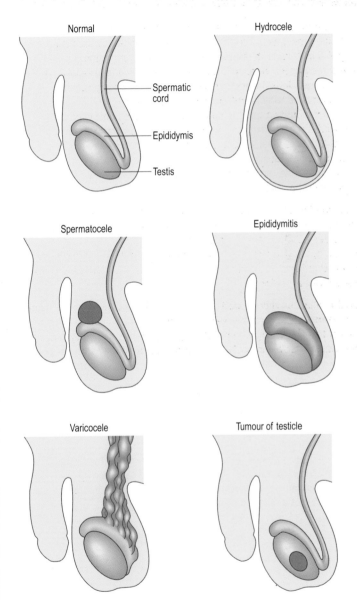

Normal

Spermatic cord

Epididymis

Testis

Hydrocele

Spermatocele

Epididymitis

Varicocele

Tumour of testicle

Fig. 6.9 Common scrotal abnormalities.

- Ask the patient to empty the bladder before the examination.
- Position the patient comfortably, either on her back or in the left lateral position with the hips and knees flexed and thighs apart.
- Use an Anglepoise lamp to illuminate the vulva adequately.
- Use gloves and lubricant gel applied to the examining fingers.
- Separate the labia minora with the forefinger and thumb of the left hand and inspect the clitoris, urethra, vagina and anus (Fig. 6.10).
- Look for any discharge, ulceration or Bartholin's gland abscesses.
- Inspect the vaginal walls for prolapse as the patient strains down and coughs; look for signs of urinary incontinence on coughing.
- Insert the index and middle fingers of the right hand into the vagina and rotate palm-upwards (Fig. 6.11). Only use one finger if vaginismus or atrophic vaginitis makes examination painful.
- Palpate the cervix: the normal cervix points downwards and slightly backwards and feels like the tip of the nose.
- Note any tenderness on moving the cervix (*cervical excitation*).
- Perform bimanual palpation: place one hand flat on the abdomen above the pubis and two fingers in the anterior fornix; identify the size, position and surface of the uterus.
- If the uterus is not palpable, palpate with the fingers in the posterior fornix as the uterus may be retroverted.
- Palpate each lateral fornix in turn bimanually.
- Note any tenderness or swelling of the *adnexa* (fallopian tubes or ovaries), the bladder anteriorly and pouch of Douglas posteriorly.

Vaginal examination is not routine but is often indicated if inflammatory or neoplastic disease of the genitourinary organs is suspected. Its intimate nature raises medicolegal considerations necessitating both informed consent and the presence of a chaperone throughout the examination.

The vaginal examination of females with an intact hymen should be avoided, particularly as the information required can often be obtained by digital examination of the rectum. Vaginal examination of minors requires the consent of a parent or guardian.

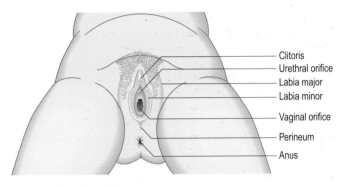

Clitoris
Urethral orifice
Labia major
Labia minor
Vaginal orifice
Perineum
Anus

Fig. 6.10 Female genital anatomy.

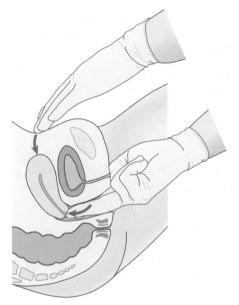

Fig. 6.11 Vaginal examination.

A

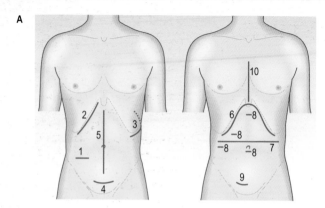

1 Lanz (appendix)
2 Kocher's (hepatobiliary)
3 Nephrectomy (extraperitoneal)
4 Pfannenstiel (gynaecology
  or caesarean section)
5 Midline

6 Roof-top (pancreatobiliary)
7 Transverse (abdominal aortic
  aneurysm, colonic surgery)
8 Laparoscopic port sites
  (for laparoscopic cholecystectomy)
9 Inguinal hernia
10 Sternotomy

B

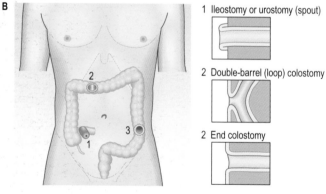

1 Ileostomy or urostomy (spout)

2 Double-barrel (loop) colostomy

2 End colostomy

Fig. 6.12   Sites of (A) scars and (B) stomas.

The neurological system

Cardinal symptoms	Stroke risk factors	Trigger factors for seizure
• Headache	• Hypertension	• Anticonvulsant withdrawal
• Dizziness	• Hyper-cholesterolaemia	• Alcohol abuse
• Blackout	• Smoking	• Sleep deprivation
• Visual disorder	• Diabetes mellitus	• Mental/physical exhaustion
• Hearing disorder	• Previous vascular event[a]	• Systemic infection
• Mental disorder	• Prosthetic heart valve	• Intracranial sepsis
• Sensory disorder	• Family history	• Metabolic disturbance
• Motor disorder	• Alcohol excess	• Dehydration
• Sphincter disorder	• Oral contraceptive pill	• Drug abuse
		• Photic stimulation

[a] Cerebrovascular accident/transient ischaemic attack/myocardial infarction/peripheral embolism

Symptom patterns and disease process

Clarify the precise meaning of patients' symptoms and the terms used to describe them. It is then often possible to make a firm diagnosis on clinical grounds alone, though confirmation may still require further investigation. The neurological history is a detailed record of the nature and course of symptoms in terms of their time-intensity relationships. The pattern of symptoms can then be interpreted within a framework of recognized stereotypes of neurological disorders. The history indicates the pathological process and physical examination its extent. For example, sudden neurological defects suggest a vascular disorder; a chronic history of relapsing symptoms with anatomically unrelated signs suggests a demyelinating disorder.

General observations – Glasgow Coma Scale, cognitive function, speech, behaviour, movement, rashes, smell of alcohol

(1) **Eyes** – Squint, ptosis, oculomotor palsies, visual acuity and fields, pupillary responses

(2) **Face** – Frontal balding, temporal arteries

(3) **Neck** – Stiffness

(4) **Abdomen** – Muscles, bladder, saddle and anal sensation

(5) **Genitalia** – Testicular atrophy

(6) **Arms and legs** – Muscles, scars, fasciculation, tone, power, reflexes, coordination, sensation, nerve root irritation

(7) **Feet** – Pes cavus, muscle wasting, trophic ulcers

Intellectual (cognitive) function

- Perform the Abbreviated Mental Test (Table 7.1) in all patients to screen for disorientation and cognitive impairment.
- Test memory by asking about both recent and distant events.
- Test attention and concentration using the 'serial sevens' test. Ask the patient to subtract 7 from 100 and to continue to subtract 7 from the remainder (normal < 1 minute with no more than two mistakes).
- Test general knowledge by asking questions about current affairs, e.g. national politics and international problems.
- Assess intelligence from patients' accounts of themselves, their occupation, ability to reason and abstract thinking. Ask the patient to explain the meaning of common proverbs such as 'a stitch in time saves nine'.

Mental state examination

- Record the appearance and demeanour of the patient; note unusual dress, mannerisms, aggression, restlessness, agitation or apathy.
- Ask about current mood and spirits. If depression is suspected, ask about biological symptoms and suicidal thoughts (Table 7.2).
- Assess the patient's speech (format, content, volume, rate of delivery).
- Assess thought by asking the patient about any intrusive thoughts, recurrent concerns or odd ideas; note the presence of any delusions.
- Ask about any unusual experiences such as hearing voices or seeing strange things (illusions and hallucinations).
- If appropriate, interview a close family member to ask about any change in mood, behaviour, personality or cognitive function.

Rapid flow of speech is typical in mania, the patient often flitting rapidly between loosely related topics '*flight of ideas*'. Both rate and volume of speech are characteristically reduced in depression.

Delusions are fixed, unshakeable unreasonable beliefs. **Hallucinations** are false perceptions (visual, auditory or tactile) in the absence of a stimulus; **illusions** are misinterpretations of normal perceptions.

7.1 Abbreviated Mental Test

(Score 1 for each correct response)

- How old are you?
- What is the time just now?
- What year is it?
- What is the name of this place? (Where are we just now?)
- Please memorize the following address: 42 West Street
- What is your birthday? (date and month)
- What year did the First World War begin?
- What is the name of the Queen?
- Can you recognize …? Two people?
- Count backwards from 20 to 1
- Repeat the address which I gave you

Normal score: 8–10

Source: Hodkinson HM 1972 Age and ageing. 1: 233–238

7.2 Biological markers of depression

Poor appetite	Sleep disturbance
Weight loss	Anhedonism
Loss of libido	Fatigue and irritability

7.3 First rank symptoms of schizophrenia

- Auditory hallucinations of following type:
  - third person
  - running commentary
  - repeating/echoing of thoughts
- Passivity of thought (withdrawal/insertion/broadcasting)
- Passivity experiences:
  - actions under external control
  - bodily sensations imposed by external agency
- Primary delusion (based on perception of everyday sight/object)

- Obtain an account from relatives, friends, neighbours or passers-by of the past medical history and events prior to clouding of consciousness.
- Check the pulse, blood pressure and respiratory rate and rhythm.
- Look for evidence of alcohol and drug abuse, skin rashes, spider naevi, hepatosplenomegaly, head injury and meningeal irritation.
- Check a bedside blood glucose measurement (BM).
- Assess changes in response to pain and verbal commands using the patient's best motor, eye and verbal responses (Glasgow Coma Scale).
- Assess pupillary diameters, symmetry and light responses.
- Look for squints, roaming eye movements and reflex eye movements on neck rotation and flexion (doll's head manoeuvre).

Coma may be defined as loss of consciousness with a Glasgow Coma Scale 3 (E1, V1, M1). It may result from structural disease of the cerebral cortex or brain stem disease (infection, stroke, haemorrhage or tumour) or metabolic disorders causing brain stem dysfunction (Tables 7.4 and 7.5).

Meningeal irritation

- Ask the patient to flex the neck, to make the chin touch the sternum.
- Place one hand beneath the occiput and rotate the head with the other hand (head jolt test); slowly flex the neck (Kernig's sign) (Fig. 7.1).
- With the patient supine and one leg extended, flex the other hip and knee to 90° and then extend the knee (Brudzinski's sign).

Meningeal irritation (*meningism*) results from inflammation of the meninges due to infection or subarachnoid bleeding, and evokes reflex spasm in the neck muscles, characterized by neck stiffness as the head is passively rotated on the cervical spine or as the neck is flexed.

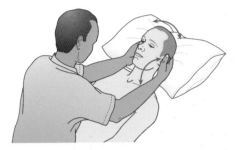

Fig. 7.1 Testing for meningeal irritation.

7.4 Metabolic causes of coma

- Hypoglycaemia
- Hypothermia
- Hyperglycaemic hyperosmolar non-ketotic states (HONK)
- Uraemia
- Hepatic encephalopathy
- Hypercapnic ventilatory failure
- Drug-induced coma (alcohol, opiates)

7.5 Glasgow Coma Scale	
Eye opening	**Score (1–4)**
Spontaneous	4
Response to speech	3
Response to pain	2
None	1
Best verbal response	**Score (1–5)**
Normal speech – oriented	5
Normal speech – disoriented	4
Inappropriate – abnormal speech	3
Incomprehensible speech	2
None	1
Best motor response	**Score (1–6)**
Obeys commands	6
Localizes to pain	5
Flexion withdrawal to pain	4
Abnormal flexion	3
Extension	2
None	1

Dysphasia, dysarthria and dysphonia (Table 7.6)

- Ask the patient to perform commands of increasing complexity, e.g. 'Close your eyes and open your mouth', and to repeat a simple sentence verbatim (*sensory or receptive dysphasia*).
- Ask the patient to identify familiar objects and then to describe everyday procedures, e.g. making a cup of tea (*motor or expressive dysphasia*).
- Ask the patient to read aloud and to vocalize labial and lingual consonants, e.g. 'British constitution', 'artillery' (*dysarthria*).
- Ask the patient to enunciate vowel sounds 'a, e, i, o, u' (*dysphonia*).
- Ask the patient to write down his or her name and address (*global language dysfunction*).

Dyspraxia (Table 7.7)

- Ask the patient to perform specific tasks, e.g. putting on spectacles.
- Ask the patient to draw figures such as squares or triangles.
- Record a sample of the patient's handwriting for later comparisons.

Cortical sensory functions (Table 7.8)

- With the patient's eyes closed, apply one or two points of the ends of a paper clip to the skin at varying distances of separation. Ask the patient to state whether one or two points are felt.
- With the patient's eyes closed, ask the patient to identify objects such as a key or a coin or pen, taking care not to make a noise.
- Ask the patient to identify unseen numbers outlined on the hand.
- Ask the patient to keep the eyes closed and to report whether sensations are felt on the right side, left side or both sides together.

NB: There is no value in testing cortical sensory functions in the presence of peripheral nerve or spinal cord sensory disorders.

7.6 Abnormalities of language and speech

- *Dysphasia* (impairment of language function from a lesion of the speech area in the dominant hemisphere) may be:
  - *expressive* (*motor*): normal understanding of speech but unable to speak the words
  - *receptive* (*sensory*): impaired understanding of speech
  - *global dysphasia*: combined receptive and expressive dysphasia
- *Dysarthria* (impairment of articulation because of defective movements of lips, tongue or palate) may be due to cerebellar disorders producing scanning or staccato speech, or disordered motor function producing slurred and indistinct speech
- *Dysphonia* (impairment of sound production) may be due to vocal cord lesions, neuromuscular weakness or extrapyramidal disorders

7.7 Dyspraxia

Difficulty in performing complex, integrated actions, e.g. lighting a cigarette or tying a shoelace, *in the absence of weakness or sensory defect*. It may be due to frontal cortex or parietal cortical dysfunction

7.8 Cortical sensory dysfunction

- *Stereognosis* – the ability to distinguish shapes, contours and textures
- *Two-point discrimination* – the ability to perceive two simultaneous stimuli as distinct when separated by minimal distances; two points on the finger tips 2–3 mm apart can normally be separated, unlike on the leg or back where the separation distance may exceed 50 mm
- *Sensory inattention* – the ability to perceive simultaneously applied stimuli at corresponding sites on both sides of the body; disordered parietal cortex function is suggested if a hemianaesthesia can only be demonstrated when stimuli are applied to both sides simultaneously but not when applied separately to either side

Olfactory nerve (I)

- Test the patency of each nostril by asking the patient to sniff, as loss of the sense of smell (*anosmia*) is commonly due to nasal disease.
- With the patient's eyes closed, ask the patient to identify common odours using an orange or tobacco.

Optic nerve (II)

Visual acuity

- Ask the patient to wear glasses if appropriate; test each eye separately.
- Test near vision by either asking the patient to read the different typefaces of a newspaper or use standard reading charts (*Jaeger card*).
- Test distant vision by reading the standard *Snellen types* at a distance of 6 metres, recording result as 6/6, 6/18, etc.

Visual fields (Figs 7.2 and 7.3)

- Sit directly opposite the patient and maintain eye-to-eye contact.
- First check for visual inattention by testing both eyes simultaneously. With arms outstretched, waggle one or both forefingers and ask the patient to report the side on which movement is observed.
- Then test each eye separately, asking the patient to cover one eye and to look into your opposing eye.

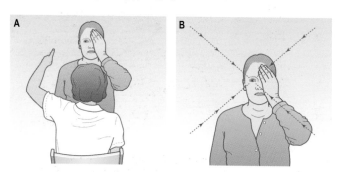

Fig. 7.2   Testing the visual fields.
(A) Position yourself in front of the patient with your outstretched finger midway between you and the patient. (B) Test each eye separately with the other eye closed. Bring the finger towards the centre of vision along diagonals drawn on an imaginary plane midway between you and the patient. Map out any defect carefully.

- Examine the outer aspects of the visual fields by waggling a finger into the field of vision from the periphery at several points on the circumference of the upper and lower, nasal and temporal quadrants.
- Ask the patient to state when the finger tip is waggling.
- Identify central field defects as the finger tip crosses the visual field.

Ophthalmoscopy

- Carefully inspect both optic fundi using the ophthalmoscope, as described on page 56.

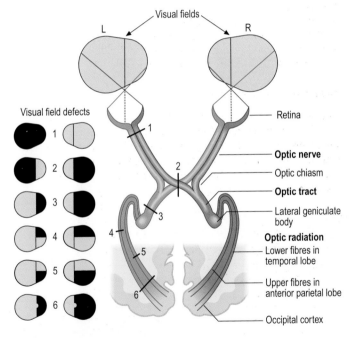

Fig. 7.3 Visual field defects.
(1) Total loss of vision in one eye because of a lesion of the optic nerve.
(2) Bitemporal hemianopia due to compression of the optic nerve. (3) Right homonymous hemianopia from a lesion of the optic tract. (4) Upper right quadrant hemianopia from a lesion of the lower fibres of the optic radiation in the temporal lobe. (5) Less commonly a lower quadrantic hemianopia occurs from a lesion of the upper fibres of the optic radiation in the anterior part of the parietal lobe.
(6) Right homonymous hemianopia with sparing of the macula due to lesion of the optic radiation in the posterior part of the parietal lobe.

Oculomotor, trochlear and abducens nerves (III, IV, VI)

Pupillary reflexes (Fig 7.4)

- Using a bright light in a darkened room, approach each eye in turn from the side; observe the direct reflex (constriction of the pupil on the stimulated side) and the consensual reflex (contralateral pupil).
- Ask the patient to gaze into the distance and then to look at the tip of the nose; observe the accommodation response of both pupils.

Ocular movements (Fig. 7.5)

- Note asymmetry of the palpebral fissures (*ptosis*) and pupil diameters.
- Look for evidence of a squint (*strabismus*): concomitant or paralytic.
- Ask the patient to watch your finger and report if double vision (*diplopia*) occurs while following the finger held at least 50 cm away.
- Move the finger up and down, both to the right and the left, noting the direction in which double vision occurs and whether the separation of the two images is horizontal, vertical or tangential.

Nystagmus

- Ask the patient to follow your finger as you move it rapidly up and down and side-to-side. Look for vertical, horizontal or rotatory oscillations.
- Note if nystagmus is jerking or pendular.
- Note the direction of gaze in which nystagmus is most marked.
- Note the direction of the fast phase of jerking nystagmus.
- Note if jerking nystagmus changes direction with the direction of gaze
- Note if nystagmus is more marked in one eye (*ataxic* or *dysconjugate nystagmus*).

Pendular nystagmus (oscillations equal in rate and amplitude) most commonly results from a defect in macular vision. *Jerking nystagmus* (oscillations with both a rapid and a slow component) may be peripheral or central in origin.

Peripheral lesions (vestibular apparatus or vestibular nerve) produce a unidirectional nystagmus irrespective of the direction of gaze. Central lesions (brain stem or cerebellum) produce bidirectional nystagmus (direction of nystagmus changes with the direction of gaze).

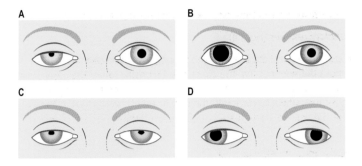

Fig. 7.4 Pupillary defects.
(A) (right) Horner's syndrome (ptosis and miosis). (B) (right) Holmes–Adie pupil. (C) Argyll Robertson pupils with bilateral ptosis and small irregular pupils. (D) III nerve palsy (looking down and out, ptosis and a dilated pupil).

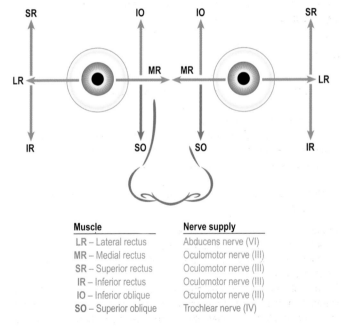

Muscle	Nerve supply
LR – Lateral rectus	Abducens nerve (VI)
MR – Medial rectus	Oculomotor nerve (III)
SR – Superior rectus	Oculomotor nerve (III)
IR – Inferior rectus	Oculomotor nerve (III)
IO – Inferior oblique	Oculomotor nerve (III)
SO – Superior oblique	Trochlear nerve (IV)

Fig. 7.5 Eye movements.
Ask the patient to cover one eye. The lateral image corresponds to the affected eye.

Trigeminal and facial nerves (V, VII)

Sensory function (V) (Fig. 7.6)

- Compare the sensations of both touch and pain in the distribution of the ophthalmic, maxillary and mandibular divisions on both sides.
- Use a wisp of cotton wool to assess the sensation in the nostrils (less distressing and easier to interpret than testing the corneal reflexes).

Motor function (V)

- Ask the patient to open the jaw against resistance; the jaw deviates towards the side of any unilateral weakness of the lateral pterygoids.
- Palpate the masseter muscles as the teeth are clenched to assess power and symmetry.
- To elicit the jaw jerk (Fig. 7.7), ask the patient to let the mouth hang open, and with a tendon hammer, strike your thumb placed on the patient's chin.

Motor function (VII) (Fig 7.8)

- Look for signs of facial paralysis: reduced wrinkling of the forehead, drooping of the corner of the mouth, flattening of the nasolabial fold.
- Ask the patient to frown and to look upwards to wrinkle the forehead; ask the patient to keep the eyes tightly shut as you try to open them.
- Ask the patient to grimace, show the teeth, and to blow out the cheeks as if trying to whistle.
- Compare upper with lower voluntary facial movements and note any differences in involuntary movements when the patient smiles.

A brisk jaw jerk suggests a bilateral upper motor neurone lesion.

Because upper facial movements on each side of the face are bilaterally innervated, unilateral upper motor neurone lesions typically reduce movements of the lower more than the upper part of the face. Lower motor neurone lesions affect upper and lower parts of the face equally.

Involuntary facial movements such as blinking, and emotional expressions such as smiling may be preserved or even exaggerated in lesions of the upper motor neurone.

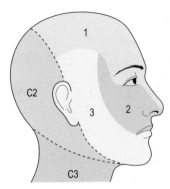

Fig. 7.6 Cutaneous distribution of the trigeminal nerve.
1, Ophthalmic division; 2, Maxillary division; 3, Mandibular division; C2, Second cervical root; C3, Third cervical root.

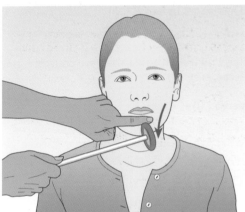

Fig. 7.7 Eliciting the jaw jerk.

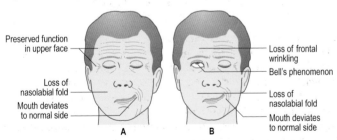

Preserved function in upper face

Loss of nasolabial fold

Mouth deviates to normal side

Loss of frontal wrinkling

Bell's phenomenon

Loss of nasolabial fold

Mouth deviates to normal side

A   B

Fig. 7.8 Types of facial weakness.
Caused in (A) by lesion of precentral area or pyramidal tract (upper motor neurone); (B) by lesion of facial nerve or nucleus (lower motor neurone), also showing Bell's phenomenon.

Vestibulocochlear nerve (VIII) (Fig. 7.9)

- Test the hearing of each ear by asking the patient to repeat numbers whispered into the ear while occluding the meatus of the opposite ear.
- *Rinne's test*: place the base of a vibrating tuning fork (256 Hz) on the mastoid bone; ask the patient to compare the sound with the sound when the other end of the vibrating tuning fork is placed at the meatus.
- *Weber's test*: Place the base of the vibrating tuning fork on the vertex of the skull and ask whether the sound is heard in the midline or preferentially in one ear.
- Inspect the external ear passages and tympanic membranes using an auriscope if hearing is impaired or if earache is a problem (p. 58).

Glossopharyngeal and vagal nerves (IX, X)

- Ask the patient to cough and to vocalize vowel sounds, 'a', 'e', 'i', 'o', 'u'.
- Observe the movements of the soft palate, uvula and posterior pharynx during the gag reflex and as the patient says 'Aaah'.

Spinal accessory nerve (XI)

- Examine the bulk of the sternocleidomastoid and trapezius muscles.
- Ask the patient to shrug both shoulders against resistance; compare the positions of each hand from behind as the patient stands with the arms by the sides (the hand hangs lower on the side of trapezius weakness).
- Test both sternocleidomastoids together by asking the patient to press the chin downwards against your hand; test each separately by asking the patient to rotate the chin to each side in turn against resistance.

Hypoglossal nerve (XII)

- Inspect the tongue in the floor of the mouth for evidence of wasting and fasciculation, then ask the patient to protrude the tongue; look for deviation to one side indicating weakness of that side of the tongue.
- Ask the patient to push the tongue against each cheek in turn while applying resistance; assess power and symmetry of movement.

Vagus nerve lesions produce dysphonia, a 'bovine' cough and failure to elevate the affected side of the soft palate. Hypoglossal nerve lesions produce wasting and fasciculation of the tongue; unilateral paralysis causes deviation of the tongue towards the paralysed side.

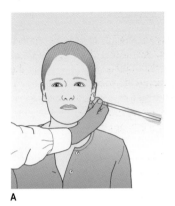

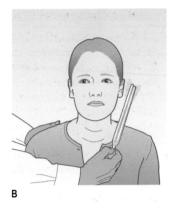

A

B

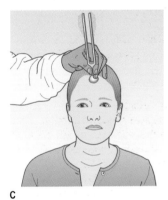

C

Fig. 7.9   Rinne's and Weber's tests.
(A and B) Rinne's test; (A) testing bone conduction; (B) testing air conduction.
(C) Weber's test.

Rinne's test   Normally, air conduction is better than bone conduction. In conduction deafness (e.g. wax build up), air conduction is reduced but bone conduction is relatively enhanced due to increased sensitivity of the auditory nerve in an attempt to overcome the defect. Thus, in conduction deafness, bone conduction will be better than air conduction, while in sensorineural deafness, air conduction will remain superior.

Weber's test   Preferential hearing of the sound in one ear indicates conductive deafness in that ear or neural deafness in the opposite ear.

133

Tremors and involuntary movements (Table 7.9)

- Ask the patient to relax in the sitting or supine position.
- Look for any tremor at rest.
- Ask the patient to stretch out the arms and look for a tremor; place a sheet of paper over the dorsum of the hands to amplify any tremor.
- Look for any involuntary movements at rest and during movement.

Muscle tone (Table 7.10)

- Ask the supine patient to relax so that the limbs are limp and floppy.
- Flex and extend the limbs at the wrists, elbows, knees and hips; manipulate each joint slowly at first and then more rapidly.
- Assess tone at the wrist by shaking the forearm and observe the floppiness of the hand.
- Assess tone at the ankle by rolling the leg to and fro (Fig. 7.10); observe the floppiness of the foot as the hip rolls from internal to external rotation.

Tremors result from alternate contraction and relaxation of groups of muscles producing rhythmic oscillations about a joint or group of joints. There are three common types of tremor

1. *Action tremor* is an exaggeration of the 10-cycles-per-second physiological tremor which underlies all apparently smooth movements. An increase in physiological tremor is often found in anxiety, hyperthyroidism and alcohol withdrawal.
2. *Resting tremor* is a coarser, slower tremor of 5 cycles per second; it is maximal at rest but absent during sleep, reduced during voluntary movement and increased by emotion. Typically it occurs in Parkinsonism, often producing adduction–abduction movements of the thumb with flexion and extension movements of the fingers.
3. *Intention tremor* is a coarse, slow tremor of 5 cycles per second, characteristic of cerebellar disorders, which is maximal during movement, present on maintaining posture and absent at rest.

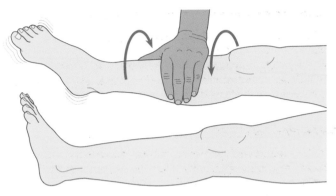

Fig. 7.10 Assessing muscle tone.

7.9 Involuntary movements

Involuntary movements (*dyskinesias*) are caused by lesions of the basal ganglia:

- *Choreiform* movements are irregular, jerky, and semi-purposive movements affecting different muscle groups unpredictably
- *Myoclonic* movements are sudden, shock-like movements of a whole limb
- *Athetoid* movements are slow, writhing movements of the distal limbs and trunk

---

7.10 Hypertonia (increased tone)

- *Spasticity* indicates pyramidal tract disorders of the upper motor neurones and produces an increasing resistance to the first few degrees of passive movement. Then, as the movement continues, there is a sudden lessening of resistance ('*clasp-knife*' *spasticity*)
- *Rigidity* indicates extrapyramidal tract disorders of the basal ganglia and produces a sustained resistance throughout the range of movement ('*lead-pipe*' *rigidity*). '*Cogwheel*' *rigidity* is the jerky resistance to passive movement seen in Parkinson's disease which results from the combination of a Parkinsonian tremor and rigidity; it is often most apparent at the wrist joint

Muscle inspection and power testing

- Record whether the patient is right- or left-handed.
- With the patient relaxed, look for muscle wasting and fasciculation; if fasciculation is suspected, tap the muscle gently with a tendon hammer to induce fasciculation.
- Assess the power in the upper limbs both proximally and distally.
- Compare one muscle group with the same group on the other side.
- Assess truncal power by asking the supine patient to touch the toes; observe any vertical or lateral movement of the umbilicus which might help to localize lesions causing muscle weakness.
- Assess the power in the lower limbs both proximally and distally.
- Compare one muscle group with the same group on the other side.

Muscle wasting is associated with physical inactivity and with myopathies; in both instances, it is typically symmetrical. Lower motor neurone lesions (denervation) produce asymmetrical wasting.

Fasciculation (visible muscle twitching) occurs randomly at rest and stops during voluntary movements; it suggests lesions in the proximal aspects of the lower motor neurones.

Muscle power

It is usually only necessary to test selective muscle groups; occasionally, however, all muscle groups require assessment. The power in the upper limbs is normally greater on the dominant side. *Isometric testing* involves the patient attempting to maintain a limb position whilst the examiner tries to move the limb. *Isotonic testing* is a more sensitive method; the patient attempts specific limb movements while the examiner opposes the movement.

7.11 Muscle groups: innervation

Movement	Muscle groups	Nerve root
Shoulder abduction	Deltoid Supraspinatus	C5, C6
Shoulder adduction	Pectoralis major Latissimus dorsi	C5–C7
Elbow flexion	Biceps, brachioradialis	C5, C6
Elbow extension	Triceps	C7
Wrist flexion	Flexor carpi ulnaris Flexor carpi radialis	C7, C8
Wrist extension	Extensor carpi ulnaris Extensor carpi radialis	C6, C7
Finger flexion	Flexor digitorum	C7, C8
Finger extension		C7
Finger abduction	Dorsal interossei	T1
Hip flexion	Iliopsoas	L1, L2
Hip extension	Gluteus maximus	L5, S1
Knee flexion	Hamstrings	S1
Knee extension	Quadriceps femoris	L3, L4
Ankle dorsiflexion	Tibialis anterior	L4
Ankle plantar flexion	Gastrocnemius	S1, S2

7.12 MRC Rating Scale for Muscle Power

Rating	
0	No visible contraction
1	Visible contraction without joint movement
2	Movement with elimination of gravity effect
3	Movement overcoming any gravity effect
4	Movement against both gravity and added resistance
5	Normal power

- Place the patient in a comfortably relaxed position to facilitate easy access to the limbs.
- Identify the tendon by palpation and then tap it with a tendon hammer, using a swinging motion from the wrist (Fig. 7.11); the tendon, not the muscle, should be struck, as stimulation of a muscle belly produces a contraction which is independent of the reflex arc.
- Compare the reflex responses on both sides, noting any delay in muscle relaxation or asymmetry of response.
- If no reflex is observed, repeat using reinforcement, always instructing the patient to relax as soon as the tendon has been struck.
- To reinforce the reflexes of the upper limbs, ask the patient to clench the jaws or squeeze the knees together just before the tendon is struck.
- To reinforce the reflexes of the lower limbs, ask the patient to lock the two hands together and to attempt to pull them apart just before the tendon is struck (*Jendrassik's manoeuvre*).
- Examine for clonus if the reflexes are brisk.

Clonus

- In a relaxed patient in the supine position with the knee extended, push the patella down briskly towards the foot to elicit knee clonus.
- With the knees flexed and the ankle in a neutral position, dorsiflex the foot briskly to elicit ankle clonus.

Disturbances of the reflexes provide strong evidence of neurological dysfunction. Upper motor neurone lesions produce pathologically brisk tendon reflexes. The absence of one or more tendon reflexes, especially if asymmetrical, denotes a lower motor neurone lesion.

Delayed muscle relaxation is characteristic of hypothermia and hypothyroidism and is often most easily demonstrable in the ankle jerk.

Clonus is the rhythmic repetition of involuntary muscular contractions evoked by a sudden passive stretch of a muscle. A few beats of clonus elicited in anxious patients may not be significant. Sustained clonus is indicative of a lesion of the upper motor neurone.

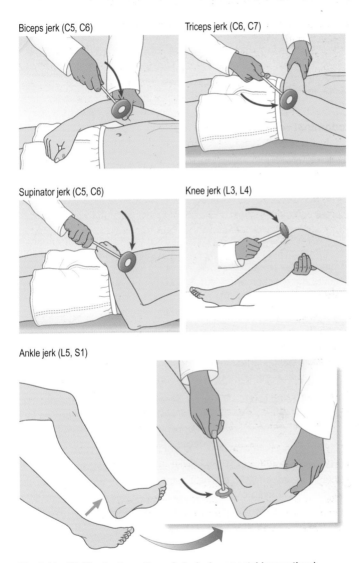

Biceps jerk (C5, C6)

Triceps jerk (C6, C7)

Supinator jerk (C5, C6)

Knee jerk (L3, L4)

Ankle jerk (L5, S1)

Fig. 7.11 Eliciting tendon reflexes (principal segmental innervations).

Hoffmann reflex (Fig. 7.12)

- Flex the distal interphalangeal joint of the patient's middle finger between finger and thumb and withdraw thumb pressure abruptly to 'flick' the distal phalanx into extension.
- Look for reflex flexion of the thumb and forefinger.

Abdominal reflexes (Fig. 7.13)

- In a relaxed, supine patient, use a blunt point to scrape the upper then lower quadrants of the abdominal wall swiftly on each side; look for reflex contraction of the abdominal wall muscles.

Plantar reflex (Fig. 7.14)

- In a relaxed, supine patient, slowly draw a blunt point, such as the tip of a thumbnail or a *Neurotip*, along the lateral border of the foot from the heel towards the little toe.
- Record the direction of the initial movement of the big toe and look for fanning of the toes. The normal response is flexion of the first metatarsophalangeal (MTP) joint; the *Babinski response* comprises extension of the big toe at the MTP joint with fanning of the other toes. Avoid undue repetition.

Hoffmann reflex is a feature of pathological hyperreflexia in the upper limbs. When present, the thumb and forefinger quickly flex in response.

Abdominal reflexes (T6–T12) may be absent if the patient has had abdominal surgery or the abdominal wall is lax. Absent responses in a young patient strongly suggest an upper motor neurone lesion for which there is usually corroborative evidence.

Plantar responses (L5, S1) may be absent if the feet are cold, or in peripheral neuropathy. An extensor plantar response (dorsiflexion of the great toe and fanning of the other toes) is due to a lesion of the upper motor neurone (*Babinski's sign*); it may be associated with reflex toe flexion on percussion of the foot's plantar surface (*Rossolimo's sign*).

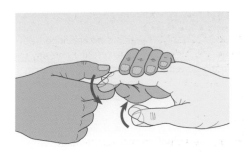

Fig. 7.12 Hoffman's sign.

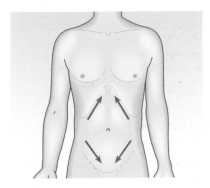

Fig. 7.13 Abdominal reflexes.

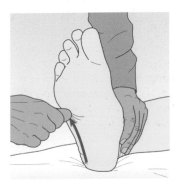

Fig. 7.14 Eliciting the plantar reflex.

Coordination

- Ask the patient to make 'piano-playing' finger movements with both arms outstretched.
- Observe the patient performing everyday activities such as fastening buttons or tying knots.
- Test rapidly alternating pronation and supination of the forearm by asking the patient to quickly slap the examiner's palm with the front and back of the hand alternately (Fig. 7.15A) (dysdiadokinesis).
- Test upper limb coordination by asking the patient to hold the arms outstretched and then to touch the tip of the nose with the tip of each index finger in turn (*finger–nose test*) (Fig. 7.15B).
- Test lower limb coordination by asking the patient to place one heel on the opposite knee and then slide the heel down the front of the shin to the ankle and back again. Repeat the test with the other heel (*heel–shin test*) (Fig. 7.15C).
- Test sitting balance with the patient's hands clasped in front.
- Test standing balance with the patient standing first with the eyes open and then with the eyes shut to assess *truncal ataxia* (*Rombergism*; p. 143).

Gait

- Observe the gait during slow and quick walking and during turns.
- Ask the patient to walk heel-to-toe along an imaginary tightrope.
- Ask the patient to hop for a short distance (cerebellar ataxia).

The smooth and accurate performance of specific movements requires intact motor, sensory and cerebellar function. Inability to perform small, precise, coordinated movements of the fingers and hands is typically found at an early stage in both pyramidal and extrapyramidal disorders.

7.13 Ataxia
Rating
<ul><li>*Sensory ataxia* (incoordination due to defective proprioception) is modified by visual feedback; ataxia is more noticeable if the patient is in the dark or has the eyes closed (*Rombergism*).</li><li>*Cerebellar ataxia* (incoordination that is unaffected by visual feedback) causes patients to 'overshoot' the target on the finger–nose test (*dysmetria*); movements are clumsy and jerky as the approach to the target is associated with an intention tremor. Rapid, alternating movements are disordered in force and rhythm (*dysdiadochokinesis*).</li></ul>

Any lesion which causes weakness may be accompanied by clumsiness but incoordination is particularly prominent in the absence of normal sensation (*sensory ataxia*) or cerebellar dysfunction (*cerebellar ataxia*).

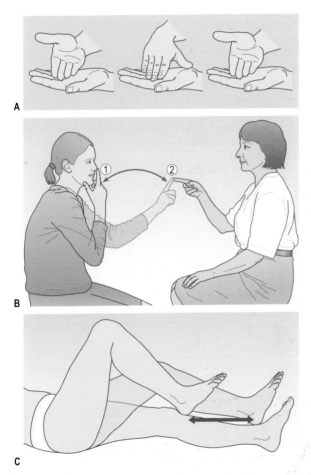

Fig. 7.15A   Testing rapid alternating movements. B. Finger–nose test. C. Heel–shin test.

Touch

- Ask the patient to keep the eyes closed and to report the touch of a point of cotton wool applied at irregular time intervals. Compare one side with the other.
- Map areas of altered sensation on the limbs or trunk, moving the stimulus from areas of diminished sensation to normal areas.

Pain

- Ask the patient to keep the eyes closed and to distinguish between the blunt and sharp ends of a pin; use a disposable Neurotip and check each dermatome as appropriate.
- Compare and contrast pain sensation between opposite sides of the body, and map areas of altered sensation.

Temperature sensation

- Test only when the other sensory modalities are unexpectedly normal (e.g. suspected *syringomyelia*).
- Ask the patient to keep the eyes closed and to distinguish between tubes containing either hot or cold water applied in a random sequence.

Localization of lesions can be deduced from an accurate interpretation of the neurological findings and a detailed knowledge of neuroanatomy (Fig. 7.16).

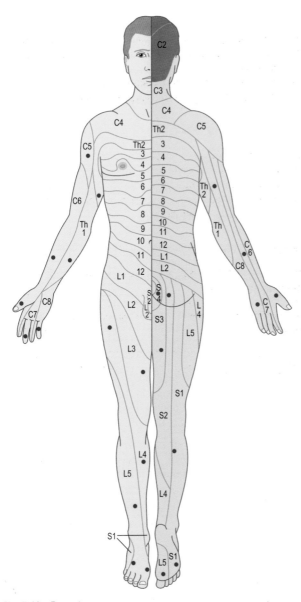

Fig. 7.16 Dermatomes.

Joint position sense

- Hold the patient's terminal phalanx with your thumb and forefinger while immobilizing the middle phalanx with your other hand.
- Flex and extend the patient's distal interphalangeal joint and ask the patient to keep the eyes closed and to indicate the directions of movement; take care to ensure that your fingers do not touch the patient's other digits.
- Look for *sensory ataxia* by testing the sitting and standing balance.

Vibration sense

- Ask the patient to describe the sensations produced by a vibrating 128 Hz tuning fork placed on the dorsum of the big toe.
- Ask the patient to report promptly when the vibration stops as you dampen the vibration.
- If vibration sense is impaired, move the tuning fork proximally to establish the level at which it is perceived.
- In the upper limbs, proceed from the distal phalanges of the fingers to the wrist and elbow.

Position and vibration sensations ascend in the ipsilateral posterior columns (Fig. 7.17); pain and temperature sensations are relayed in the posterior horns and cross to form the spinothalamic tract on the opposite side.

Joint position sense impairment usually affects the distal parts of the limbs first; testing individual joint movements therefore should begin with the fingers and toes. Only if joint position sense is impaired peripherally need similar tests be employed more proximally.

Loss of balance is suggested from the history; difficulty in walking in the dark or with eyes closed suggests sensory ataxia (Rombergism) but difficulty in walking with the eyes open suggests cerebellar ataxia.

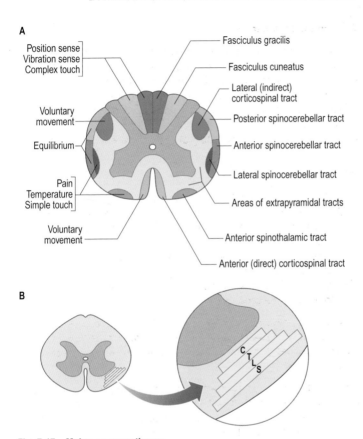

Fig. 7.17 Main sensory pathways.
(A) Cross-section of the thoracic spinal cord. (B) Distribution of spinotholamic tracts at the cervical level. Cervical segments (C) lie centrally, with the thoracic (T), lumbar (L) and sacral segments (S) lying progressively more laterally.

Sciatic nerve roots (Fig. 7.18A and B)

- Position the patient supine and slowly flex the hip with the knee fully extended to stretch the nerve roots.
- Ask the patient to report any pain as soon as it is experienced and to indicate the site of the pain.
- Look for tenderness over the sciatic nerve by compressing the mid-buttock over the greater sciatic notch.

Femoral nerve roots (Fig. 7.18C and D)

- Position the patient prone and slowly extend the hip with the knee flexed to 90°.
- Ask the patient to report any pain as soon as it is experienced and to indicate the site of the pain.

When lumbar nerve roots are compressed, e.g. prolapsed intervertebral disc, stretching of the affected nerve gives rise to pain in the lower back and/or buttock radiating into the leg.

Sciatic nerve roots are tested by hip flexion (straight leg raising). Normally, 90° of pain-free hip flexion should be possible; compression produces pain radiating from the back down the back of the leg to the foot.

Femoral nerve roots are tested by hip extension; compression causes pain radiating from the back down the front of the leg to the knee and limitation of hip extension.

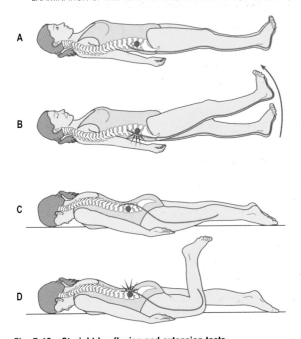

Fig. 7.18 Straight leg flexion and extension tests.
(A and B) Stretch test – sciatic nerve roots: (A) neutral; nerve roots slack; (B) straight leg raising limited by tension of root over prolapsed disc. (C and D) Stretch test – femoral nerve: (C) patient prone and free from pain because femoral roots are slack; (D) when femoral roots are tightened by extension of the hip, pain may be felt in the back.

Features of upper motor neurone (pyramidal tract) lesions

- Paresis or paralysis
- Hypertonia of spastic type
- Increased tendon reflexes and clonus
- Absence of cutaneous reflexes
- An extensor plantar response

Features of lower motor neurone lesions

- Paresis or paralysis
- Hypotonia
- Muscle wasting
- Muscle fasciculation
- Diminished or absent tendon reflexes

Features of cerebellar lesions

- Limb ataxia
- Truncal ataxia
- Intention tremor
- Jerking nystagmus (bidirectional)
- Scanning dysarthria

Features of mixed sensorimotor polyneuropathies

- Impaired sensation affecting all modalities
- Sensory loss occurring in a 'stocking' ± 'glove' distribution
- Muscle wasting and fasciculation, particularly in the distal limbs
- Muscle weakness, particularly of distal limb movements
- Diminished or absent tendon reflexes

Features of posterior column lesions (ipsilateral)

- Sensory ataxia of the limbs
- Preservation of pain and temperature sensations
- Impaired joint position sense
- Impaired vibration sense
- Preservation of the tendon reflexes

Features of spinothalamic tract lesions (contralateral)

- Dissociate sensory loss with selective impairment of pain and temperature sensation and preservation of vibration, touch and joint position sense
- Loss of tendon reflexes
- Preservation of motor function

Features of extrinsic spinal cord lesions

- Early radicular pain and localized spinal tenderness
- Preservation of perineal sensation (sacral sparing)
- Loss of sensation over many dermatomes
- Progression to sphincter disturbance
- Spastic paresis or paralysis

Features of intrinsic spinal cord lesions

- Late development of pain or spinal tenderness
- Loss of perineal sensation (saddle anaesthesia)
- Dissociate sensory loss (selective loss of pain sensation)
- Early onset of sphincter dysfunction
- Spastic paresis or paralysis

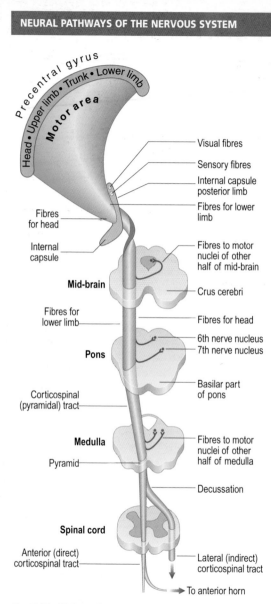

Fig. 7.19   Motor pathways.

The locomotor system

Cardinal symptoms	Extra-articular features	Functional assessment
• Joint pain	• Fever and night sweats	• Washing/toileting
• Joint stiffness	• Rashes/gouty tophi/RA nodules	• Getting dressed
• Joint swelling	• Raynaud's/nail dystrophy	• Holding a pen/spoon
• Weakness	• Dry/red/painful eyes	• Opening cans/bottles
• Hot/red joint(s)	• Dry mouth/mouth ulcers	• Climbing stairs
• Loss of function	• Diarrhoea/urethritis	• Employment status

8.1 Patterns of joint disease	
Monoarticular	Septic arthritis, trauma, crystal arthritis (gout), haemarthrosis
Oligoarticular	
Non-inflammatory	Osteoarthritis (OA) (especially large joints)
Inflammatory	Ankylosing spondylitis, reactive arthritis, psoriasis, polymyalgia rheumatica
Polyarticular	
Non-inflammatory	Pain and stiffness worse on activity, improved by rest
	Typically affects weight-bearing (large) joints and only slowly progressive
Inflammatory	Pain and stiffness: worse on resting, improved by activity
Flitting pattern	Resolves in one joint and moves to another (rheumatic fever)
Additive pattern	Affects an increasing number of joints (rheumatoid arthritis)
Symmetrical	Typically non-weight-bearing joints: rheumatoid arthritis (RA), systemic lupus erythematosus (SLE), juvenile chronic arthritis (JCA)
Asymmetrical	Typically lower limb joints: ankylosing spondylitis, psoriasis, reactive arthritis, gout (history of previous acute attacks), pseudogout

General observations – Nutrition, walking and other aids, demeanour, po[sture,] functional ability

(1) **Hands and arms** – RA nodules, nails, joint swelling

(2) **Eyes and face** – Anaemia, scleritis, iritis

(3) **Head and neck** – SLE rash, cranial arteries, goitre, lymph nodes, psoriasis, gouty tophi (pinnas)

(4) **Chest** – Pleurisy, pericarditis

(5) **Abdomen** – Splenomegaly

(6) **Genitalia** – Balanitis, Reiter's disease

(7) **Legs and feet** – Swelling, deformity, plantar fasciitis, gouty tophi

Look – Joint deformities, swellings, scars, muscle wasting, skin changes, limb lengths

Feel – Tenderness over joint lines, tendons, bursae, ligaments, warmth, swelling, joint effusions

Move – Range of active and passive movements, crepitus, ligament integrity, fixed flexion deformities, muscle weakness, Trendelenburg sign

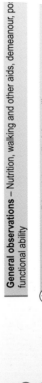

EXAMINATION OF THE HAND JOINTS

General principles

- Check active movements before passive if arthritis is painful.
- Measure and record the range of movements of important joints.
- If active movements are normal, avoid testing passive movements.

Look

- Inspect the joints of the hands and wrists: with the patient seated, compare the two sides; note the symmetry of joint involvement, swollen joints or tendon sheath abnormalities.
- Look for ulnar drift of the fingers at the metacarpophalangeal (MCP) joints (partial subluxation) and wrist joints (carpal subluxation) seen in RA (Fig. 8.1). Also look for spindling of the fingers and small bony lumps at the proximal interphalangeal (PIP) joints (*Bouchard's nodes*) and the distal interphalangeal (DIP) joints (*Heberden's nodes*) seen in OA.
- Look for joint deformities: *'swan neck'*, *'boutonnière'*, *'trigger finger'* and *'mallet finger'* deformities of the fingers in RA (Fig. 8.1).

Feel

- Palpate the joint margins of the wrists, MCP, PIP and DIP joints. Note any thickening of the palmar fascia (*Dupuytren's contracture*).

Move

- Assess active movements: ask the patient to clench the fists, show the palms, touch the little finger with the thumb and put the wrists through a full range of movements.
- Check for triggering of the fingers: ask the patient to make and release a fist quickly. Tendon sheath thickening may prevent the straightening of the fingers. If triggering of a finger is present, feel the tendon sheath in the palm of the hand as the patient attempts extension.
- Check ulnar and median nerve function: the median nerve supplies the intrinsic muscles of the thenar eminence (unable to abduct thumb against resistance) and the ulnar nerve supplies most of the intrinsic muscles of the hand (unable to adduct fingers). For sensation see Figure 8.2.
- Assess passive movements: identify the nature of any limitation of movements of the small joints of the hand and wrists.
- Feel for crepitus in the small joints of the hands and wrists as you take the hand and wrist joints through a full range of movements.

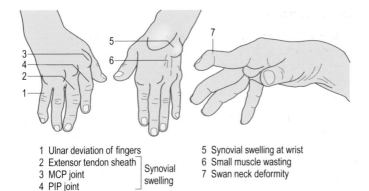

1 Ulnar deviation of fingers
2 Extensor tendon sheath ⎤
3 MCP joint   ⎥ Synovial
4 PIP joint   ⎦ swelling
5 Synovial swelling at wrist
6 Small muscle wasting
7 Swan neck deformity

Fig. 8.1   Arthritic changes in the hand in rheumatoid arthritis.

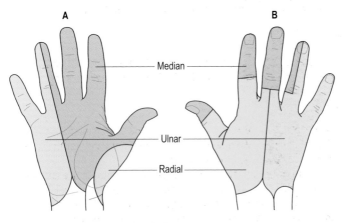

Fig. 8.2   Sensory innervation of the hand.
(A) Anterior view. (B) Posterior view.

Look

- Inspect the shoulders: compare both shoulders, note any postural change, swelling, scars, muscle wasting, 'winging' of the scapula (long thoracic nerve palsy).

Feel

- Palpate the joint margins: look for signs of swelling, redness or heat.

Move

- Assess shoulder function: ask the patient to touch the back of the head with both hands and then to place both hands behind the back, to try to touch the shoulder blades (Fig. 8.3A,B).
- Assess glenohumeral joint rotation: with the arm in 90° flexion at the elbow, ask the patient to rotate the arm and shoulder internally and externally; note any pain or limitation (Fig. 8.3C).
- Assess abduction and adduction of the shoulder: place one hand on the scapula to assess movement attributable to the scapula rather than the glenohumeral joint, note any pain or limitation in the arc of movement from adduction to full abduction (normal 180°) (Fig. 8.3D).
- Assess flexion and extension of the shoulder: stabilize the scapula with one hand and ask the patient to move the arm from full flexion to extension (normal 180°) (Fig. 8.3E).

Other tests

- Test for a painful arc: passively abduct the arm through an arc of 180°; note the point at which pain is experienced. In a rotator cuff injury, the transition from 120° to 40° is painful (Fig. 8.3F,G).
- Test the integrity of the supraspinatus tendon: ask the patient to abduct the arm starting with the arm against the side. Supraspinatus tendon rupture prevents the patient initiating the first 30° of active abduction of the arm, but the patient may achieve full abduction if assisted by passive abduction through the first 30°.

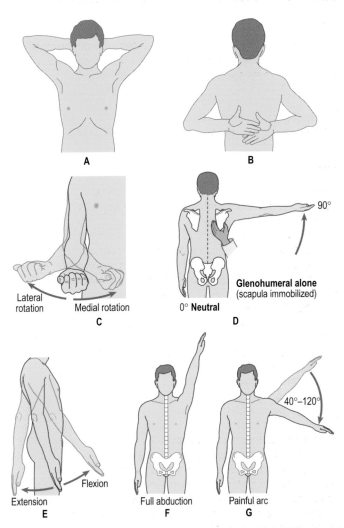

Fig. 8.3A–G (A,B) Positions for overall function of the shoulder. (C) Degrees of glenohumeral rotation. (D) Abduction/adduction with scapular stabilization. (E) Degree of flexion/extension at the shoulder joint. (F,G) Painful arc syndrome.

Look

- Assess the gait: look specifically for a limp and a Trendelenburg gait.
- Inspect the affected joint: with the patient standing, compare both hips, note any swelling, scars and gluteal muscle wasting. Ask the patient to lift one leg off the floor and look for pelvic tilting (*Trendelenburg's sign*).
- Measure the true and apparent leg lengths: true leg length is measured from the anterior superior iliac crest and apparent leg length from the umbilicus (Fig. 8.4).

Feel

- Palpate over the hip joint: note any areas of tenderness.

Move

- Test for fixed hip flexion (*Thomas's test*): in the supine patient with knee extended, place one hand beneath the lumbar spine and elevate each leg in turn to the point at which the lumbar lordosis disappears. If fixed flexion is present, the opposite leg will rise off the bed (Fig. 8.5).
- Flexion and extension of each hip: in the supine patient with knee flexed, elevate the leg towards the abdomen; with the patient standing, draw the leg backwards.
- Abduction and adduction of each hip: in the supine patient, place your arm across the pelvis to assess any movement due to pelvic tilting, and move each leg in turn from full abduction (45°) to full adduction (25°). Note any limitation or pain (Fig. 8.6A).
- Internal and external rotation of each hip: in the supine patient, flex the hip to 90° and using the lower leg, assess the range of rotation – normally 30° of internal rotation and 45° of external rotation (Fig. 8.6B).
- Look for evidence of sacroiliitis: with the patient lying supine, compress the pelvic girdle by leaning firmly on both anterior iliac crests; alternatively, roll the patient into the left lateral position to compress the pelvic girdle by leaning firmly on the right anterior iliac crest. In patients with seronegative, spondyloarthritis, stressing the sacroiliac joints will cause discomfort if there is active sacroiliitis.

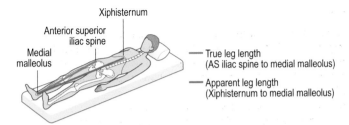

Fig. 8.4 Apparent and true leg length.

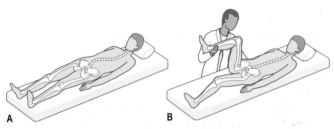

Fig. 8.5 Flexion deformity of the left hip (Thomas's hip flexion test).
Full flexion of the right hip reveals the flexion deformity on the left side.

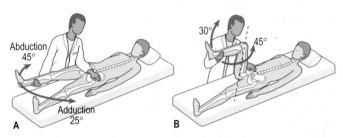

Fig. 8.6 Testing (A) adduction/abduction and (B) internal/external rotation of the hip joint.

Look

- Inspect the joint: with the patient lying supine, compare both knees; note any swelling, scars, quadriceps muscle wasting, effusions, ankle oedema.
- Ask the patient to stand: assess any angulation of the knee joint (*varus* = knock-kneed; *valgus* = bow-legged).

Feel

- Palpate the joint margins: ask the patient to partially flex the knee and palpate the joint line, medial and lateral collateral ligaments and the site of insertion of the patellar tendon; note any swelling or tenderness. Feel in the popliteal fossa for the presence of a Baker's cyst.
- Test for an effusion: use the patellar tap and massage tests (Figs 8.7 and 8.8).

Move

- Assess active movements: ask the patient to fully flex the knee, then to extend the knee fully by pushing your hand into the bed with the knee. The normal range of movement is 0–140°.
- Assess passive movements: lift the leg with one hand on the ankle and the other under the thigh; assess the range of flexion and extension.
- Feel for crepitus at the knee and the patellofemoral joints; feel the knee as it is being flexed; feel the patella as it is moved over the femoral condyles.

Other tests

- Test the stability of the knee: assess the medial and lateral collateral ligaments by checking the laxity on lateral and medial flexion of the lower limb with the leg straight. Assess the cruciate ligaments by checking the anteroposterior (AP) laxity of the semi-flexed knee, rocking the tibia to and fro while immobilizing the foot by sitting on it (Fig. 8.9).
- Test meniscal integrity: hold the ankle and slowly extend the flexed knee with the knee internally rotated; repeat with the knee externally rotated. A positive result produces a palpable clunk and patient discomfort (*McMurray's test*). Alternatively, ask the patient to squat from a standing position.

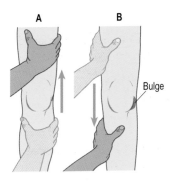

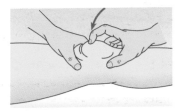

Fig. 8.7 Testing for an effusion in the right knee by the massage test. (A) Massage any fluid away from the side of the knee. (B) Apply firm downward pressure over the lateral side of the knee and observe for fluid displacement.

Fig. 8.8 Testing for an effusion by the patellar tap test.

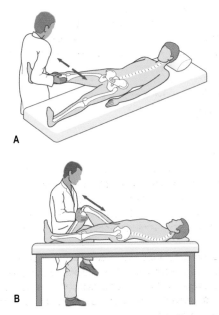

Fig. 8.9 Testing (A) the collateral and (B) the cruciate ligaments of the knee.

Cervical spine

- Look for abnormal posture or swellings, from the front, back and sides.
- Feel for tenderness over the bony prominences and paraspinal muscles.
- Assess movement at the neck: rotation, lateral flexion and AP flexion/extension (Fig. 8.10).
- Examine the upper limbs neurologically.

Thoracic spine

- Look for abnormal posture (kyphosis/scoliosis) from the back and side.
- Feel for tenderness over the bony prominences and paraspinal muscles.
- Assess movement at the thoracic spine: rotation and AP flexion/extension with the patient seated.
- Measure chest expansion: normal 5 cm or more.

Lumbar spine

- Look for abnormal posture (scoliosis/loss of lordosis), from the back and side, with the patient standing.
- Feel for tenderness over the bony prominences and paraspinal muscles.
- Assess movement at the lumbar spine through AP and lateral flexion/extension (Fig. 8.11).
- Assess spinal flexion using *Schober's test* (Fig. 8.12): locate the line between the posterior superior iliac crests (L3/4 interspace); mark two points 10 cm above and 5 cm below this line. Ask the patient to bend forward as far as possible, with the knees extended. The two points separate by 5+ cm on flexion in health and < 5 cm in ankylosing spondylitis.
- Tests for prolapsed lumbar disc nerve root compression: (p. 148). Straight leg flexion to 90° in the supine patient should be pain-free; in L4/L5/S1 nerve root compression, flexion is limited by pain radiating down the back of the leg to the foot (pain increased by dorsiflexing the ankle, *Bragaard's test*). In L2/L3/L4 nerve root compression, straight leg extension produces pain down the front of the leg to the knee.

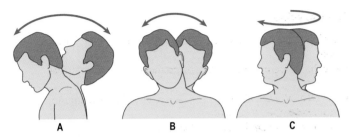

Fig. 8.10 Cervical movements.
(A) Flexion/extension. (B) Lateral flexion. (C) Rotation.

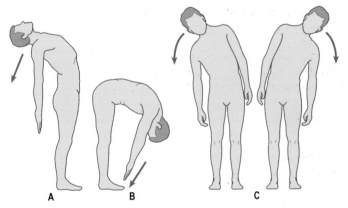

Fig. 8.11 Movements of the spine.
(A) Extension. (B) Flexion. (C) Lateral flexion.

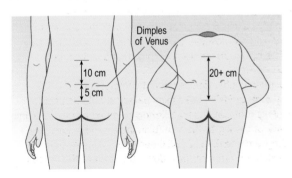

Fig. 8.12 Schober's test of spinal flexion.

- Observe the posture: a stooped and round-shouldered appearance suggests vertebral osteoporosis with kyphosis (Fig. 8.13).
- Observe the gait: ask the patient to take 10 steps and then return. Note if the balance is disturbed during the turn. A slow shuffling gait suggests Parkinsonism or cerebral atherosclerosis; a broad-based gait, truncal ataxia (cerebellar disease); and a high-stepping gait, foot drop.
- Look for evidence of a spastic gait: note if the patient abducts one leg more than the other when walking, scuffing one shoe with each step, indicating a hemiplegia (Fig. 8.14).
- Ask the patient to stand on one leg then the other: note if additional support (or a walking stick) is required to perform this manoeuvre; inability to weight-bear even with support is strong evidence of a femoral fracture or septic arthritis of the hip or knee.
- Look for evidence of a painful abnormality of the gait: note if one limb is flexed with the foot placed delicately on the floor for as little time as possible to avoid the pain of weight-bearing, indicating sciatica or a painful hip, knee or ankle.
- Look for evidence of a painless abnormality of the gait: the *waddling gait* or *Trendelenburg gait* is characteristic of patients with bilateral, congenital dislocation of the hips or gluteal abductor muscle weakness, e.g. osteomalacia or muscular dystrophy.

A painful gait produces a '*dot–dash, dot–dash*' pattern (the shorter pause (dot) on the painful limb and the longer pause (dash) on the painless limb).

Shortening of one leg from surgery, deformity or joint stiffness disturbs the normal smooth rhythm of the gait causing a painless limp (*dash–dot, dash–dot*) with the longer pause on the abnormal limb.

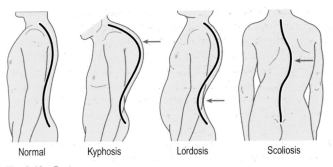

| Normal | Kyphosis | Lordosis | Scoliosis |

Fig. 8.13   Posture.

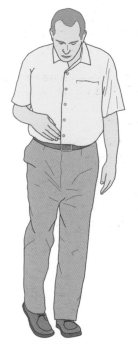

Hemiplegic gait
- leg stiffness
- forced flexion of foot
- hip adduction
- knee extension

Fig. 8.14   Hemiplegic gait.

The critically ill patient

9

- Rapidly check that the patient is conscious, has a pulse and is breathing with a patent airway. If the patient is not breathing and/or pulseless, call for help immediately and start basic life support (BLS) (Table 9.1).
- Assess the level of consciousness using the AVPU system (Tables 9.2 and 9.3): if head injury or stroke is suspected, also record the Glasgow Coma Scale (GCS; p.123).
- If unresponsive or responding only to pain, recheck ABC – airway, breathing, circulation – check blood glucose and secure intravenous (IV) access.
- If responsive, take a brief history of the presenting complaints.
- Record the respiratory rate (RR): if > 24 breaths per minute, reassess the patient and check oximetry.
- Check oximetry: if oxygen saturation < 93%, check the oximeter probe position before checking arterial blood gases, then administer oxygen therapy.
- Record the heart rate (HR): if rate < 40 or > 110 beats per minute, check the ECG, reassess the patient, place on a cardiac monitor and secure IV access.
- Record the blood pressure (BP): if the systolic BP < 100 mmHg, check the BP manually, secure IV access and consider an IV fluid challenge. Monitor the HR, BP, RR and hourly urine output (catheterize if in doubt) (Table 9.4).
- Check the capillary filling time: gently depress a fingernail or toenail until it blanches and record the time taken for the colour to return (normally < 2 seconds).
- Check the patient's temperature: if 38°C+ or < 36°C, check blood, urine and sputum cultures and consider antibiotic therapy as appropriate.
- Review all the patient's recent drug therapy.
- If the patient is stable, take a detailed history and examine all systems.
- Call a senior colleague for assistance if in any doubt.

Patients admitted to intensive care units (ICU) are often inadequately assessed or monitored prior to admission to the ICU. Use of an early warning system (EWS) to identify and monitor patients at risk of rapid clinical deterioration should help to avert potentially avoidable disasters.

9.1 Adult basic life support algorithm

Check responsiveness	Check safety of rescuer/victim
	Shake and shout, 'Are you alright?'
	No response? Shout for help!
Open airway	Head tilt
	Chin lift
Check breathing	Look at chest wall
(10 seconds)	Listen at mouth
	Feel for air on your cheek
	No response? Go for help
Breathe	Give 2 effective breaths
Assess circulation	Check carotid pulse?
(10 seconds)	Look for signs of circulation:
	swallowing?
	breathing?
	movements?
If the circulation is Present	Continue rescue breathing at 10 per minute
	Check circulation every minute
If the circulation is Absent	Start chest compressions at 100 per minute
	Combine compressions: rescue breathing
	Ratio = 15 compressions : 2 breaths

9.2 Early warning system (EWS) checklist

- Neurological status
- Respiratory rate
- Heart rate
- Blood pressure
- Temperature
- Oximetry
- Blood glucose

9.3 Neurological status: AVPU system

- **A**lert – the patient is alert and oriented in time and place
- **V**erbal – includes the patient who is asleep or confused
- **P**ain – check the GCS if the patient only responds to pain
- **U**nresponsive – seek expert help immediately

9.4 Peripheral circulatory failure – 'shock'

- Tissue turgor – evidence of water depletion
- Capillary filling time – normally < 2 s: 3+ s in 'shock'
- Postural hypotension – BP supine > BP erect
- Systolic BP < 100 mmHg
- Tachycardia – HR > 100 b.p.m.
- Urine output < 30 mL/h for 3 consecutive hours

Index

173